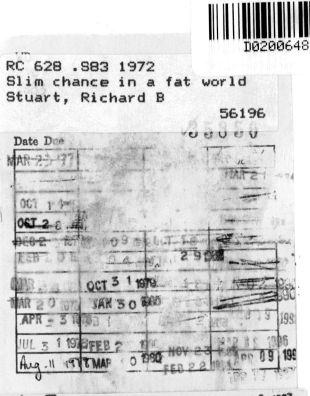

SLIM CHANCE
IN A FAT WORLD:

BEHAVIORAL CONTROL OF OBESITY

Richard B. Stuart
Barbara Davis

Research Press
2612 North Mattis Avenue
Champaign, Illinois 61820

To our two spouses and six children
who all but gave up hope of
seeing us again for a time.

CONTENTS

ACKNOWLEDGMENTS

Many writers have contributed to the development of the ideas presented in this book, but several scientists stand out as having had a profound influence upon the shaping of the concepts of obesity and its management as represented here. These giants in their fields are Sir Stanley Davidson, Dr. J.V.G.A. Durnin, Dr. Jean Mayer, Dr. R. Passmore, Dr. Stanley Schachter, and Dr. Albert J. Stunkard. To these men we wish to extend our respectful thanks.

In addition, the authors wish to express their deep gratitude to Dr. Frances Larkin, of the University of Michigan School of Public Health, for her critical review of sections of the manuscript; to Mrs. Dorothy Caputi for her expert medical illustration of the text; and to Miss Noni Lipson and Mrs. Loraine Reish for their work in the preparation of the manuscript. Finally we wish to express our boundless thanks to Miss Lynn Nilles whose sanity was tried many times as she was called upon to help us express our ideas in an intelligible manner and to provide continuity to a manuscript by authors with "distinctive" styles.

FOREWORD

This book is the best guide to weight reduction to appear so far. It makes available to the general public, for the first time, the results of a remarkable recent surge of interest in the treatment of obesity. It describes the techniques of behavior modification which, for the past four years, have been applied with considerable success to this widespread and stubborn disorder.

What is behavior modification? Also known as behavior therapy, it is an attempt to correct disorders of human behavior by applying principles of learning discovered in the laboratory. Originally these techniques were used to treat alcoholism and phobias. But there is mounting evidence that behavior modification is more effective than traditional methods in a variety of disorders. Its application to the treatment of obesity is a late development, but a fruitful one.

Until quite recently, many professionals took a pessimistic view of the obese individual's chances of controlling his weight. I summed up this attitude a few years ago in saying that "Most obese persons will not remain in treatment. Of those who do remain in treatment, most will not lose much weight, and of those who do lose weight, most will regain it." More concretely, a review of treatment results reported in the medical literature revealed that only 25% of persons who entered treatment for obesity lost as much as 20 pounds, and only 5% lost as much as 40 pounds.

Some of the prevailing gloom suddenly lifted when, in 1967, a small journal devoted to behavior modification research published a short paper by Richard Stuart titled, "Behavioral Control of Overeating." In it, the author described the best results ever obtained in office treatment of obesity. Of eight persons who remained in treatment (even Stuart lost two of his original ten), *all* lost more than 20 pounds, and three lost more than 40 pounds. The report had an electrifying effect on researchers working in this field, and sparked a series of other trials of behavior therapy in obesity.

This surge of interest produced vast amounts of data. I know of no area of psychological treatment that has turned up so much information so rapidly. To date, at least nine studies have been undertaken to compare the effectiveness of behavior modification to that of traditional methods used to treat various kinds of obese persons. In an unusual display of unanimity, each of these studies has found behavior modification to be the most effective treatment method. Until now, trials have been limited to carefully selected groups of overweight persons, treated on an experimental basis. With the publication of *Slim Chance,* behavior modification methods become available to a wider audience.

The authors have wisely included three vitally important elements in their program: behavioral control of eating, management of food intake, and management of exercise. Any comprehensive weight control program requires all three. But the unique and imaginative element here is, of course, behavioral control of eating. Here is something every overweight individual can read to great advantage. He may well find, as I did, some of his own favorite weight control maneuvers described. If so, the theoretical explanation for their usefulness may be of great value, showing him how he can adopt similar maneuvers described in the book, and how he can devise new ones along the same lines. The section on food intake is an excellent review of information that we often know about and seldom use. The authors offer a number of ingenious suggestions to help the reader make better use of what he has learned about eating.

The section on exercise, or management of energy expenditure, is particularly timely. The authors call to our attention an important and under-recognized discovery of the noted nutritionist Jean Mayer. Dr. Mayer has exploded the myth that exercise merely increases food intake. He found that when many sedentary persons increase their physical activity, they actually eat less. This double benefit of exercise—increasing calories burned, decreasing calories consumed—has been ignored for too long. Just this year, the importance of exercise to successful reducing was highlighted in a weight reducing program conducted at Chicago's Michael Reese Hospital. Dr. William Shipman, the program's director, found that exercise made the difference: Only those persons who increased their physical activity lost weight.

There are those who will wonder whether behavior modification, however successful in the experimental treatment situation, can really be achieved through the medium of a book. Most veterans of the weight reduction wars have already tried books as they have tried diets, drugs, and reducing machines—all to no avail. Beyond its short-term inspirational effect, can a book really help anyone lose weight?

Until recently, most psychiatrists would have said "no." It has long been an article of faith in psychotherapy that enduring changes in human behavior can be achieved only with the help of a personal relationship. But now this traditional idea has been challenged. Dr. Richard Hagen, of Florida State University, has shown that a group of overweight women who used a behavior modification manual lost as much weight as another group treated by therapists using this same manual. This surprising effectiveness of "therapy without a therapist" has yet to be confirmed by other investigators.

Whether the readers of *Slim Chance* will be able to use this volume as effectively as Dr. Hagen's fortunate patients used their manual is a question each reader will have to answer for himself. But when the going gets tough, it may help to know that it has been done.

Anyone who has ever tried to lose weight knows that the road is rough. This book is no short cut. If your weight problem is purely cosmetic, you may be willing to make the effort necessary to achieve a slimmer, more attractive figure. Or you may not. Are the cosmetic benefits, appealing as they may be, worth the extensive changes in your pattern of daily living that the program requires? For many, the answer may well be "no."

But this program has implications that go beyond obesity control. As serious as the problem of obesity is in its own right, its twin causes—increased food intake and diminished physical activity—are even more serious from a medical standpoint, for both play a role in the development of coronary artery disease, which is now, by a wide margin, the leading cause of death in this country. Measures designed to control eating, guarantee proper food selection, and increase physical activity may not only help control obesity but may also help prevent coronary artery disease.

Slim Chance calls for a great deal of hard work. This program is likely to be more successful than those that have preceded it, but it won't be any easier. In fact, it will be harder. And the effort required must be continued over many months and even years, until changes in eating and exercise become second nature. Despite its advantages, behavior modification is no panacea. But in a sense, the demands of the program are the key to success. Earlier weight reduction programs asked only that one suffer and endure; this one provides the opportunity to work hard and succeed. And herein lies its attraction. Its carefully designed, step-wise progress toward active mastery of a problem can lead not only to the control of obesity, but also to a more rewarding, inner-directed life.

Albert J. Stunkard, M.D.
6 October 1971

Chapter 1

THE WHAT, WHO, AND HOW OF OBESITY, AND WHAT SHOULD BE DONE ABOUT IT

Obesity has been "the companion of mankind"[1] for over 12,000 years as evidenced by the plump figure of the "Venus of Willendorf," a small carving dating from the Stone Age. Obesity has risen and fallen as a function of social customs, declining in the days of the Old Testament when the scriptures forbade the eating of animal fat, rising with the gluttony of the Roman Empire, and undulating thereafter as a function of richness or poverty in what Wyden has not so facetiously termed the "thorn of plenty."[2] At the present time it is estimated that there are some 40 to 80 million obese Americans, depending upon the criteria used. Furthermore, despite warnings by the prestigious Public Health Service that obesity "is one of the most prevalent health problems in the United States today"[3] and by noted English authorities such as Dr. I. McLean Baird that "obesity is one of the cardinal challenges of our times,"[4] the spread of obesity continues unabated.

There are two interrelated explanations for the growth of obesity as a public health problem. First, the eating habits of children and adults in the developed countries have changed radically during the recent past. Dr. George Christakis, former Director of the New York City Bureau of Nutrition, has suggested that nutritionists' zeal to improve contemporary eating habits has been one source of the problem.[5] He noted that following the discovery of vitamins and amino acids during the third and fourth decades of this century, nutritionists undertook broad community educational programs to spread the consumption of foods rich in both nutrients. Regrettably they did not educate as vigorously that it is essential to reduce the consumption of other foods while increasing the amounts of vitamin- and protein-rich foodstuffs. And this unfortunately occurred at a time when eating assumed a recreational character to an unprecedented extent — with the rise of cookouts, TV snacks, coffee breaks, and dinner parties, all associated with increased expendable income — and when new convenience foods flooded the market in ever-more-enticing packages. As eating habits have changed, so too have the patterns of energy use — with the family's second car replacing the walk to the school bus which earlier replaced the bicycle and, before it, the walk to school, and with the effortless washer-dryer replacing the wringer-washer which earlier displaced the scrub board. As energy use at home and at work has fallen and as food intake has increased, belts have inevitably been loosened around the waists of people of all ages. As girths expand, the immediate and delayed, inconvenient and grave consequences of obesity are felt. Not only does obesity frequently lead to embarrassment, an inability to participate in many pleasurable activities, and a lack of opportunity for social and occupational success, but it also often interferes with the simplest daily tasks such as dressing or self-care activities while exposing the obese person to heightened risk of incapacitating illnesses.

With women being more attuned to their weight problems than men,[6] the menace of obesity has reached a high level of awareness among Americans. Wyden reported that a poll conducted by the Alfred Politz Research Company in 1964 showed that:

> ... some 9.5 million said that they were on diets, another 16.5 million reported that they were watching their weight so they wouldn't gain, and still another 26.1 million expressed some concern about their waistlines. It was reasonable to conclude, therefore, that the ranks of the calorie-conscious added up to fifty-two million eaters.[7]

These calorie-counting, weight-watching, pill-swallowing masses have hung upon every word uttered by competent nutritionists and food faddists alike. MacLeod candidly noted in 1957:

> The poor nutritionist can hardly open his mouth without making the headlines as the advocate of a new dietary religion. Few sciences have suffered more from popular acclaim.[8]

If the nutritional scientists have suffered, the purveyors of gimmicks and miracle foods have prospered. Dr. Joseph Fee and his colleagues found that only one segment of the diet food industry achieved sales of $150,000,000 within two years of the introduction of "liquid meals" for dieters, while sales of appetite suppressants reached $80,000,000.[9] Regrettably much of the energy spent in the watching of waistlines and much of the money spent on food substitutes and appetite suppressants appears to be wasted as the proportion of the population which is obese is stable if not growing slightly.

WHAT IS OBESITY?

While it is generally recognized that the prevalence of obesity and its seriousness make it a major public health problem, there is little general agreement as to a precise means for determining exactly who is obese.

While obesity is regarded as a condition involving an excessive proportion of fat or adipose tissue in the body mass, some fat is essential for human survival. Not only does fat provide protection for other tissue and organs but it also performs chemical transformations analogous to those performed by the liver.[10] Estimates of the percent of fat in "normal" body composition are still speculative, but best estimates show that women are better endowed with adiposity than men and that the percent of body mass in fat tissue increases as a function of age (see Table 1).

TABLE 1

PERCENT OF WEIGHT OF SUBCUTANEOUS FAT IN TOTAL WEIGHT BY AGE AND SEX, ESTIMATED FOR PERSONS OF "STANDARD" WEIGHT FOR HEIGHT

| Age | Estimated Percent of Total Body Weight | | | |
| | Men | | Women | |
	Keys[a]	USPHS[b]	Keys	USPHS
25	14	13	26	26
35		17		30
45		22		34
50	35		43	
55		26		38

a. Keys, A., Body composition and its change with age and diet. In E. S. Eppright, P. Swanson, and C. A. Iverson (Eds.), *Weight Control.* Ames, Iowa: Iowa State College Press, 1955. P. 22.
b. U. S. Public Health Service. *Skinfolds, body girths, biacromial diameter, and selected anthropometric indices of adults: United States, 1960-62.* Washington, D.C.: U. S. Government Printing Office, 1970.

A number of different means have been used to determine the presence of obesity, some simpler and some more valid than others.[11] Arranged in order of increasing sophistication, the following list identifies some of the methods commonly encountered:

1. Surface measures
   a. The "mirror" test — identification of a "fat" appearance when an individual views himself standing nude before a mirror;
   b. The "twist" test — twisting rapidly while nude and observing whether the superficial fat tissue moves in concert with the underlying tissue;
   c. The "ruler" test — determining whether the line running from the rib cage to the pelvis is flat or concave when a ruler is placed upon the area while lying flat (indicating no obesity).

2. Anthropometric measures
   a. The "belt" test — determining whether the circumference of the chest, at the level of the nipples, is greater than the circumference of the waist at the level of the navel;
   b. The "magic 36" test — determining whether the waist girth in inches, subtracted from the height in inches, yields a number greater than 36 (indicating no obesity);
   c. Reference to tables of average or desirable weight (see the following section);
   d. The Ponderal index — determining whether the height in inches divided by the cube root of the weight in pounds yields a number greater than 12 (indicating no obesity).

3. Measurement of fat as a percentage of body weight
   a. The "pinch" test — determining whether the density of skin pinched at various body points is greater or less than one-half inch;
   b. Measurement of skinfold density using constant-tension calipers (see section on skinfold measurement);
   c. Chemical and physical measurement techniques such as densitometry, isotope dilution, measurements of exchangeable electrolyte, gamma emission of K^{40} from the body, radiography, and hydrometry.

Clearly the two most commonly used measures of obesity are reference to height/weight tables and skinfold measurement of fat mass. Accordingly, each of these techniques will be discussed in detail.

Tables of height/weight. Tables of average weight have been available in the United States since 1912 and have been updated in 1929, 1943, 1959, and 1965.[12] The first two sessions were based upon the weight and height of men and women of various ages. Unfortunately these widely used tables were limited by the fact that the 200,000 or so persons whose dimensions they reflected were not representative of the general population, as all were insurance policyholders or applicants and hence were probably members of middle and upper socioeconomic groups. A second weakness in these tables was the fact that they reflected a rise in weight with age, unintentionally implying that maturity-onset obesity was, if not desirable, at least acceptable. Therefore several improvements were undertaken in the tables constructed in 1943 and 1959. While still based upon data obtained from insurance policyholders, the age distribution was replaced with designation of desirable weights for men and women of differing height and frame size, as determined from the actuarial experience of the insurance writers. While considered an improvement over

4

their predecessors, these tables did not provide adequate guidelines for differentiating between small, medium, and large builds nor did they standardize the conditions of weighing, so that estimated nude weights for men and women were believed to be eight and five pounds less than the tabular weights respectively.

The last major weight and height survey was undertaken by the Health Examination Survey Unit of the United States Public Health Service.[13] The survey examined a randomly selected national sample of 6,672 persons between the ages of 18 and 79 from October, 1959 through December, 1962. These data indicated that men reached their maximum average weight of 172 pounds between the ages of 35 and 54 while women reached their maximum average weight of 152 pounds in the 55 to 64 year range. Following the attainment of peak weights, both sexes dropped in average weight, men falling to an average of 150 pounds and women to an average of 138 pounds during the 75 to 79 year bracket (see Figure 1). Interestingly, the heights of both men and women are also lower during the advanced states of life than during the "prime of life" (see Figure 2). Explanations for the fact that weights and heights diminish as a function of age are varied. Height may decrease because of an "inability to maintain

FIGURE 1

AVERAGE WEIGHT IN POUNDS FOR ADULTS, 18-79 YEARS

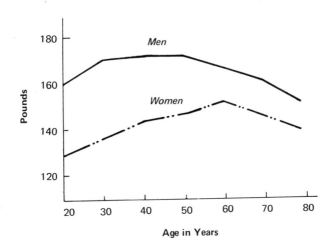

From U.S. Public Health Service, *Weight, height, and selected body dimensions of adults: United States, 1960-1962.* Washington, D.C.: U.S. Government Printing Office, 1965, P. 7.

erect posture, compression of the spinal column, and various forms of arthritis."[14] Weight decreases may be related to secular trends which favor increasing weight during middle age and the preferential survival of smaller persons at advanced age.

As an indication of secular trends, Karpinos'[15] data revealed that inductees into the military in 1957-58 were, on the average, 1.17 inches taller and 17.7 pounds heavier than inductees into service during World War I. Another secular trend favoring the gradual growth of average stature may be found in genetic changes associated with the interbreeding of persons with different geographic origins. Just as horticulturists have

FIGURE 2

AVERAGE HEIGHT IN INCHES FROM ADULTS, 18-79 YEARS

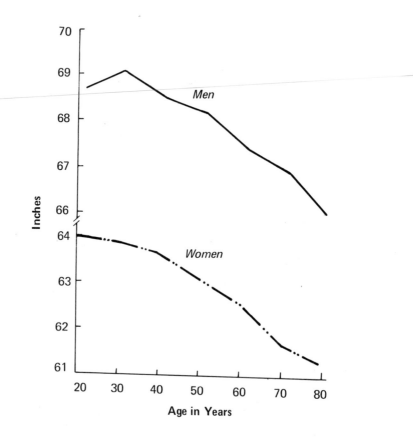

From U.S. Public Health Service, *Weight, height, and selected body dimensions of adults: United States, 1960-1962.* Washington, D.C.: U.S. Government Printing Office, 1965. P. 9.

identified the process of heterosis or hybrid vigor associated with cross-breeding,[16] human geneticists may find similar effects among humans who have never before had the opportunity to go so far afield in such large numbers to select mates.

Another conclusion which can be drawn from the height and weight data pertains to the differential survival of the sexes. Despite the fact that women tend to be heavier — relative to their mean weights at 18 to 24 years — at advancing ages, women also have differentially greater expectancies. As can be seen in Table 2, in each year since 1900 the life expectancy of women has exceeded that of men for whites and nonwhites alike, with the average woman being expected to outlive the average man by 7.3 years in 1968. Therefore it is clear that, for reasons yet unknown, men are far more sensitive to changes associated with aging than women, with body weight seeming to be a major factor.

Finally, when the data collected by the United States Public Health Service are compared with the standards developed by the Society of Actuaries,[17] it can be shown that 35 percent of all American men and 40 percent of all American women 40 years and over are at least 20 percent overweight. Comparable estimates have also been made for the English adult population, where best estimates indicate that 60 percent of the men and 53 percent of the women between 40 and 49 years of age are found to be significantly overweight.[18] In interpreting these data, however,

TABLE 2

EXPECTATION OF LIFE AT BIRTH IN THE UNITED STATES

(Years)

YEAR	White			Nonwhite			All Races		
	Male	Female	Total	Male	Female	Total	Male	Female	Total
1900	46.6	48.7	47.6	32.5	33.5	33.0	46.3	48.3	47.3
1910	48.6	52.0	50.3	33.8	37.5	35.6	48.4	51.8	50.0
1920	54.4	55.6	54.9	45.5	45.2	45.3	53.6	54.6	54.1
1930	59.7	63.5	61.4	47.3	49.2	48.1	58.1	61.6	59.7
1940	62.1	66.6	64.2	51.5	54.9	53.1	60.8	65.2	62.9
1950	66.5	72.2	69.1	59.1	62.9	60.8	65.6	71.1	68.2
1955	67.4	73.7	70.5	61.4	66.1	63.7	66.7	72.8	69.6
1960	67.4	74.1	70.6	61.1	66.3	63.6	66.6	73.1	69.7
1961	67.8	74.5	71.0	61.9	67.0	64.4	67.0	73.6	70.2
1962	67.6	74.4	70.9	61.5	66.8	64.1	66.8	73.4	70.0
1963	67.5	74.4	70.8	60.9	66.5	63.6	66.6	73.4	69.9
1964	67.7	74.6	71.0	61.1	67.2	64.1	66.9	73.7	70.2
1965	67.6	74.7	71.0	61.1	67.4	64.1	66.8	73.7	70.2
1966	67.6	74.7	71.0	60.7	67.4	64.0	66.7	73.8	70.1
1967	67.8	75.1	71.3	61.1	68.2	64.6	67.0	74.2	70.5
1968	67.6	74.9	71.1	60.3	67.6	63.9	66.7	74.0	70.2

From *National Center for Health Statistics, U. S. Department of Health, Education, and Welfare. The data for 1968 are preliminary.*

considerable caution is needed, for overweight is not isotonic with obesity. In fact, as will be shown below, the correlation between weight and more direct measures of obesity is close but not always consistent. Therefore, the Public Health Service has cautioned:

> It cannot be overstressed that assigning a label of obese to any one person or group of persons should come only after a comprehensive assessment of all pertinent factors. The sex of the subject, age, body type, and state of health, along with specific measurements such as skinfold thickness, must be considered in determining if a person is obese. Comparing any individual or group in terms of their heights and weights with a given set of averages or standards does *not* give adequate information on which to assess obesity since such comparisons imply *weight* not *fatness.* [19]

Skinfold Measurement. Drs. Carl Seltzer and Jean Mayer[20] of the Harvard University School of Public Health have noted that obesity (excessive fatness) may not be at all consistent with overweight (weight in excess of average). They suggest, for example, that:

> College football linemen are generally overweight; they are generally not obese. Conversely, some extremely sedentary persons can be obese without being markedly overweight.[21]

In their judgment, skinfold measurement is a better means of assessing obesity than weight. Skinfold measurements have been in use since 1921[22] and have been practical since the invention of constant-tension calipers by Franzen in 1929.[23] Skinfold measurements may be taken with the use of external calipers (exerting constant pressure of 10 gm. per sq. mm. with a contact surface of 20 to 40 sq. mm.) to measure skinfolds in certain areas of the body. The triceps skinfold is a highly reliable means of assessing the density of the 50 percent of total adiposity or fat tissue which is situated just under the skin. The procedure for taking skinfold measurements is described by Mayer in the following way:

> The person making the measurement pinches up a full fold of skin and subcutaneous tissue with the thumb and forefinger of his left hand at a distance about 1 cm. from the site at which the calipers are to be placed, pulling the fold away from the underlying muscle. The fold is pinched up firmly and held while the measurement is being taken. The calipers are applied to the fold about 1 cm. below the fingers, so that the pressure on the fold at the point measured is exerted by the faces of the caliper and not by the fingers. The handle of the caliper is released to permit the full force of the caliper arm pressure; and the dial is read to the nearest 0.5 mm. Caliper application should be made at least twice for stable readings. If the folds are extremely thick, dial readings should be made three seconds after applying caliper pressure.[24]

Mayer suggests that the triceps skinfold, measured at exactly one half of the distance between the shoulder and elbow, may be the easiest and most representative of the available sites, with other sites being found in the subscapular, abdominal, hip, pectoral, and calf areas.

The National Health Survey of the United States Public Health Service has included skinfold measurements as one of its indices of assessment. Data produced by this survey indicate that the average right arm skinfold density for American men is 1.3 centimeters as compared with a density of 2.2 centimeters for women. Further, as can be seen in

FIGURE 3
AVERAGE RIGHT-ARM SKINFOLD FOR ADULTS, 18-79 YEARS

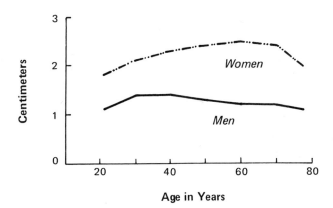

From U. S. Public Health Service, *Skinfolds, body girths, biacromial diameter, and selected anthropometric indices of adults: United States, 1960-62.* Washington, D.C.: U. S. Government Printing Office, 1970. P. 6.

Figure 3, age changes were slight for men and moderate for women, with the values for both groups being comparable at early and late adult ages.

Using the triceps skinfold measurement, Seltzer and Mayer[25] suggest that skinfold densities greater than one standard deviation above the mean (below which would fall approximately 84 percent of the population) would constitute obesity. Figure 4 and Table 3, reprinted with the permission of Drs. Seltzer and Mayer, indicate the lower limits of obesity for Caucasian Americans as derived from their research.

While techniques such as densimetric, hydrometric, and whole-body potassium measurement may be more precise,[26] skinfold measurement appears to be a more than adequately sensitive measure of obesity. Garn,

FIGURE 4

LOWER LIMITS OF OBESITY FOR CAUCASIAN AMERICANS
BASED ON MEASUREMENTS OF SKINFOLD THICKNESS

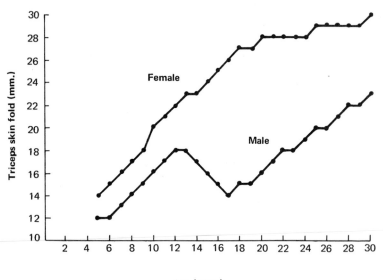

Age (years)

Reproduced with permission from C. C. Seltzer and J. Mayer, A simple criterion of obesity. *Postgraduate Medicine*, 1965, *38*, A-106.

Rosen, and McCann[27] have correlated the weight and triceps skin measurements of 359 Michigan adults and 1,099 Michigan adolescents. They show correlations of 0.52 and above for all groups except white male adults (0.36) and Negro male adults (0.44). With these values it is clear that skinfold and weight are not perfectly coincidental, but it is also clear that skinfold measurements have strong face validity as determined by their association with gross body weight.

Because skinfold measurement is relatively insensitive to the daily-weekly-monthly bodily changes which provide essential feedback about the effectiveness of a person's weight-reducing regimen, it is essential to supplement skinfold measurements with weight as determined by a balance-bar scale at the same time each day, preferably morning or evening without clothes. Moreover, it is essential to record these weights graphically in order to convey visual meaning to any changes.

WHO ARE THE OBESE?

It should be clear from the foregoing section that estimates of the number of obese persons lack precision because of their use of imprecise techniques of measurement and their dependence on assessment of differing indices of obesity. Nevertheless it is possible to discuss with some confidence the characteristics of groups having differentially high and low risk of obesity. These groups can be identified by their age, sex, socioeconomic status, cultural identification, and family characteristics.

TABLE 3

OBESITY STANDARDS IN CAUCASIAN AMERICANS

AGE (years)	MINIMUM TRICEPS SKINFOLD THICKNESS INDICATING OBESITY (millimeters)	
	Males	Females
5	12	14
6	12	15
7	13	16
8	14	17
9	15	18
10	16	20
11	17	21
12	18	22
13	18	23
14	17	23
15	16	24
16	15	25
17	14	26
18	15	27
19	15	27
20	16	28
21	17	28
22	18	28
23	18	28
24	19	28
25	20	29
26	20	29
27	21	29
28	22	29
29	22	29
30-50	23	30

Reproduced with permission from C. C. Seltzer and J. Mayer, A simple criterion of obesity, *Postgraduate Medicine*, 1965, *38*, A-105.

Age. The National Health Survey has shown that men and women tend to reach their maximum weights at about the ages of 40 and 60 respectively, with gradual weight loss being seen in later life.[28] Therefore, using weight as a parameter, middle age appears to be the most problematic time for maturation-related obesity. When waist girth is considered, a somewhat different pattern appears. The average man in the National Survey measured 35.0 inches at the waist compared with the average woman whose waist girth was 30.2 inches.[29] As can be seen in Figure 5, however, the rate of gain in waist girth averaged 4.7 inches for men between 20 and 60, declining moderately (0.9 inches) through the age of 75 to 79. In contrast, women gained consistently, averaging a gain of 2.9 inches until the age of 75 to 79, at which time there is a slight loss (0.3) registered. The increase in waist girth associated with a decrease in gross weight may be a consequence of a general "settling" of posture as reflected in a decrease in height. However it is more likely to be an indication of a trend toward

FIGURE 5
AVERAGE WAIST GIRTH FOR ADULTS, 18-79 YEARS

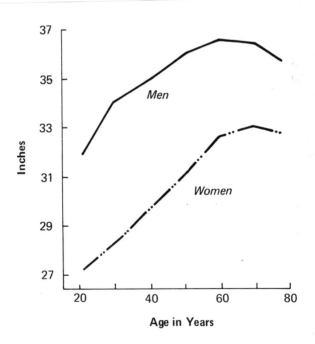

From U. S. Public Health Service, *Skinfolds, body girths, biacromial diameter, and selected anthropometric indices of adults: United States, 1960-62.* Washington, D.C.: U. S. Government Printing Office, 1970. P. 21.

FIGURE 6
RELATIVE CHANGE IN WEIGHT WITH AGE OVER THE
MEAN FOR MEN AND WOMEN AGED 18-24 YEARS

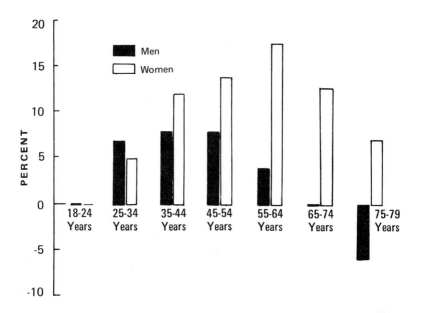

From U. S. Public Health Service, *Weight, height, and selected body dimensions of adults: United States, 1960-62.* Washington, D.C.: U. S. Government Printing Office, 1965. P. 7.

obesity when it is viewed in the light of the increase in skinfold density seen in Figure 3. The fact that weight and skinfold density both decline during the most advanced ages is probably a reflection of the operation of a process of selective survival favoring the longevity of nonobese persons.[30] Therefore it can be said that older persons have a greater risk of obesity, and it is prudent from a life-sustaining point of view for middle and older age persons to be particularly concerned about the signs of obesity.

Sex. The data summarized in Figures 1, 3, and 5 all show a trend toward obesity among men during their late twenties and thirties and among women during their forties and fifties. Thus while obese men outnumber obese women during the early adult years, obese women outnumber obese men during the later stages of adulthood. These relationships are vividly seen in Figure 6. This shows that while the longevity of women seems to be moderately influenced by obesity — the percent of overweight in women surviving to 75 to 79 years being slightly greater than that of women in the 25 to 34 year age range — the longevity of men is dramatically correlated with the percent of overweight. Men who survive to the range of 55 to 64 show a lower degree of overweight than was evident during the 25 to 34 year range, while average weight appears to be associated with survival to the 65 to 74 year range and mild underaverage weight with survival to the 75 to 79 range.

Socioeconomic status. The prevalence of obesity among different age and sex groups is complicated by the influence of additional factors including socioeconomic status, cultural factors, and family characteristics. Socioeconomic status refers to the social class of an individual or family and is commonly measured by taking a composite of factors such as the total family income, the area of residence of the family within a city of known characteristics, the rest of the family's housing, the education of the adults, and the profession(s) of the breadwinner(s). The study that provided the most frequently quoted data relating obesity with socioeconomic status is the Midtown Manhattan Study[31] which, under the general directorship of Dr. Lee Srole, randomly sampled from census tract data 1,660 adults residing in New York City. Essentially undertaken to ascertain mental health needs in the community, Dr. Srole and his associates included in their research an assessment of the occurrence of obesity, these data having been analyzed under the separate authorship of Drs. Goldblatt, Moore, and Stunkard.[32] The data show a clear inverse relationship between the prevalence of obesity and social class, that is, the lower the social class the higher the probability of obesity. Specifically, the study revealed that 32 percent of the men and 30 percent of the women in the lower socioeconomic group were obese in contrast with 16 percent of the men and 5 percent of the women in the upper socioeconomic group. Furthermore, the data indicate that obesity was more probable among downwardly socially mobile (22 percent) than among upwardly socially mobile (12 percent) individuals.

Beyond predicting obesity, social class can also be a predictor of thinness and dieting. Dr. Goldblatt and his associates found that, at least for women, increasing status was associated with a trend toward thinness. For men, on the other hand, increasing status was associated with a trend toward "normal" weight. Specifically:

> . . . there were four times as many thin respondents among women of high status as there were among those of low status. Among men, however, about 10% were thin in all classes, and it was the percentage of normal-weight respondents that increased with increasing status.[33]

Moreover, several recent studies have shown that a higher proportion of upper- as opposed to lower-class persons are concerned with or are presently following some dietary regimen.[34] For example, Wyden[35] showed that while 11 percent of the national population falls within the upper socioeconomic group, one fourth of the dieters belong to this group. Therefore socioeconomic status may effectively predict not only obesity and thinness but also the likelihood that action will be taken to correct obesity.

While a full explanation of this association between obesity and socioeconomic status awaits documentation, several plausible explanations may be offered. First, it is possible that poverty may be for obesity what ragweed is for hay fever — a pathogen subtly present but not detected because of the greater prominence of other cues. By this it is suggested that poverty may lead to poor education (including education about health and nutrition), little access to the opportunity for vigorous exercise, and proscription from those aspects of the occupational hierarchy which differentially reward nonobese persons. Second, it is possible that lower socioecnonmic groups may place a positive value upon obesity either as a means of survival,[36] as an aesthetic trait, or as a countercultural or at least subcultural norm. This would imply that, denied access to the requisites of a sound diet, occupants of lower socioeconomic strata might place a positive value upon obesity as a sign of rejection of middle-class values, a possibility which finds some support in the fact that the dominant American reference groups do seem to regard obesity as a form of social deviance.[37]

Ethnic factors. Dr. Goldblatt and his associates have observed that "obesity may in part depend on social status, but, at the same time, social status may in part depend on obesity."[38] Ethnic or cultural factors are another contributor to obesity and may, in fact, constrain the rise of an obese person up the socioeconomic ladder. The anthropologist who is concerned with the study of ethnic variables is interested in the values which guide behavior and which serve to evaluate an action which has occurred. Ethnic variables can be shown to govern a wide variety of the conditions associated with eating, ranging from the delineation of times when it is appropriate to eat and the selection of edible substances, to the means of food preparation and the ceremony associated with eating, among others. For example, Brown has demonstrated that:

> Food can be defined as an objectively edible substance, that is, one that is capable of nourishing the body, but edible substances must be culturally defined as food before they will be eaten. Thus what we eat is in large measure determined by the culture in which we live and to some degree by our economic and status position within the society.[39]

The basis for these culturally governed decisions about the acceptability of food leaves much to be desired, often being highly illogical. For example, as late as 1954 the anthropologist Titiev noted that:

> There is no society known, including our own, which has first made a thorough scientific analysis of all the nutritive elements in the environment, and then given items preference in the order that they were known to be best suited to man's biological needs. Instead, ethnologists found everywhere the existence of food preferences based upon artificial, man-made values, that have little or nothing to do with nutrition as such.[40]

While plant foods are eaten selectively in each culture, it has been suggested that "most culturally banned foods to which particular revulsion attaches are of animal origin."[41] As but one example, Professor Dorothy Lee noted:

> We do not recognize dragon-flies as human food; the Ifugao do. They eat three species of dragon-fly, as well as locusts which are boiled, then dried, then powdered and stored for food. They eat crickets and flying ants which they fry in lard. They eat red ants and water bugs and a variety of beetles. I doubt that I would recognize these insects as food, however hungry I might be. On the other hand, I regard milk as food, a fluid which some cultural groups regard with disgust and as akin to a mucous discharge.[42]

One need not venture as far as the Ifugao culture of the Philippine Islands, however, to find the influence of cultural factors upon food selection. For example, for those Americans of Mexican origin chili and beans are staples while other Americans of corresponding education and income levels regard these foods as cocktail party rarities; the chitlins and grits common in the diets of southeastern Americans are not found in the diets of persons living in other regions; and potatoes are considered to be an appropriate and common side dish for breakfast eggs within but not beyond a belt of states stretching from the American Southeast to the Rocky Mountains. Finally, with respect to the values associated with body build, Drs. Dwyer, Feldman, and Mayer have noted:

> Just as fashions in clothes vary, norms and ideals for bodily appearance change from culture to culture and over time. Arabs, for example, esteem different, plumper body types than do Americans. During the late Renaissance, a young woman who had wide hips and an ample expanse of abdomen regarded herself as beautiful, while her twentieth-century American counterpart abhors these very characteristics in herself. Thus, since norms and ideals do change, there is no reason to assume that the current ones will last forever. Slimness may remain in vogue [in middle- and upper-class America], or it may be replaced by a more amply padded figure. Such shifts could have striking prevalence of concern over weight and on dieting efforts.[43]

TABLE 4
DISTRIBUTION OF OBESITY AMONG NINE ETHNIC GROUPS
(WOMEN)

Ethnic Group	Socioeconomic Status	Total	% Obese
American (fourth generation)	low	15	13
	medium	23	4
	high	102	4
Puerto Rican	low	13	15
	medium	4	25
	high	1	0
Russian, Polish, Lithuanian	low	11	18
	medium	25	12
	high	41	10
British	low	13	23
	medium	22	0
	high	21	10
Irish	low	69	25
	medium	51	16
	high	29	3
Italian	low	31	32
	medium	31	23
	high	5	20
German, Austrian	low	82	35
	medium	69	16
	high	55	4
Czech	low	46	41
	medium	17	29
	high	5	0
Hungarian	low	16	44
	medium	17	24
	high	11	0

Reproduced with permission from A.J. Stunkard, Environment and obesity: Recent advances in our understanding of regulation of food intake in man. *Federation Proceedings*, 1968, 27, 1369.

As a validation in fact of what theory tells us might be true about the association between ethnic orientation and obesity, Drs. Goldblatt, Moore, and Stunkard[44] showed that first-generation women were almost five times as likely to be obese as fourth-generation women (24 as opposed to 5 percent) while the same ratio appears to hold for men, of whom approximately 32 percent were obese in the first generation as opposed to approximately 8 percent in the fourth generation. (It should be added that the authors also found a statistically significant relationship between generation in the United States and socioeconomic class, the lower socioeconomic status positions tending to be associated with recency of immigration.) Furthermore, Dr. Stunkard has recently released additional, previously unpublished data from this investigation (see Table 4).[45] Shown as an interaction between ethnic identification and socioeconomic status, this table reveals that the percentage of obese women varies widely across different ethnic groupings. For example, in contrast to lower-class fourth-generation Americans, 13 percent of whom were obese, 44 percent of the lower-status first-generation Hungarians studied were obese. While the sample sizes in this study are small relative to the population — e.g., a total of 825 women participating in this phase of the study from a total city population of over 7,000,000 — there is no obvious reason for supposing that the relationship between the obtained values for each subsample would have varied had the sample size been larger.

Familial factors. If the forces of culture are found to leave their indelible imprint upon all aspects of individual behavior ranging from food choice to the value placed upon body build, then the effects of family interaction can be expected to be even more sharply focused. Yet there are some curious inconsistencies. For example, while husbands and wives eat as many as 18 out of 21 meals in common weekly over a 20-year period, there are low-order similarities between the caloric value of diets of the weight profiles of husbands and wives.[46] The correlation between the number of kilocalories per day for husbands and wives was found, among 104 pairs, to be only .445 while the husband-wife similarities in alcoholic beverage consumption reached .785.[47] In contrast, the parent-child similarities in body build and diet are higher than would be expected by chance, with some indicators suggesting a greater mother-child than father-child similarity.[48] As these similarities extend as well to sibling-sibling comparisons, one might suppose that some combination of genetic and environmental factors might account for obesity. However Garn[49] analyzed data which show that there is a decreasing resemblance of siblings in later life and further that the adult differences in monozygetic twins and triplets are so great as to create serious question about the validity of the genetic hypothesis. He suggests:

> There is genetic control of fat patterning, there may be genetic control of relative fatness, but since twins who cease to eat together then diminish their fat resemblances, the genetic hypothesis for obesity is less tenable than that of the home environment.[50]

Some evidence for the specific interactions in the home environment which bears upon patterns of eating has been collected in unpublished research by Stuart. He arranged for the dinner-table verbal interaction between women who were clients in a weight reduction program and their husbands to be recorded on thirty-minute audio casette tapes. Coding certain interactional variables from the tapes indicated:

1. Husbands were seven times more likely than their weight-reducing wives to initiate food relevant topics of conversation;

18

2. Husbands were almost four times more likely than their wives to proffer food to the spouse;

3. Wives were slightly over twice as likely as their husbands to reject food offers; and

4. Husbands were over twelve times as likely to offer criticism of their wives' eating behavior than they were to praise it.

Several problems have so far prevented the publication of these data. The first is sample size, data being available from only fourteen couples. The second is the problem of representativeness — only three tapes being available from each couple. Finally, a means has not yet been devised for determining precisely whether the criticized eating of the wife did in fact involve an inappropriate food choice.

Nevertheless, the data so far available did appear to warrant the collection of data pertaining to husbands' attitudes toward their wives' body size. Clinical interviews with fifty-five husbands of overweight women are revealed in Table 5. To the extent that these data reflect salient food-related exchanges between spouses, it should be clear that some, although by no means all, husbands of obese wives are not only not

TABLE 5
HUSBANDS' ATTITUDES TOWARDS WEIGHT LOSS BY WIVES

1. Do you wish to see your wife lose weight?
Yes	50
No	3
Don't care	2

2. Are you willing to assist your wife in losing weight?
Yes	27
No	17
Did not answer	11

3. Is your wife heavier now than when you married?
Yes	41
No	8
Same	6

4. In your own words, what changes would weight reduction by your wife mean to you?*
Loss of eating as a shared activity	29
Loss of bargaining position in arguments	27
Fear of losing wife in divorce	21
Increased worry of wife's unfaithfulness	17

*These data were coded from free response answers and do not include answers offered by less than one-fifth of the respondents. Each respondent offered an average of 3.1 responses in the six blanks available.

contributors to their wives' efforts to lose weight, but they may actually exert a negative influence. Because of weaknesses in the sampling and data-collection procedures, it would be hazardous to generalize specific findings beyond the families directly involved in this study, but the data would seem to support the inferences that the influence mediated by husbands over the eating behavior of their wives is subtle, found in apparently inconsequential verbal exchanges, and quite profound.

What is true for husband-wife interactions is even more likely to characterize the parent-child interactions, and therefore Garn seems well-justified in asserting that the "key person in obesity appears to be the mother, or mother-surrogate . . . who has the keys to the cupboard, and can be the 'pusher' . . . of calories."[51] Indeed it defies the imagination to conceive of an obese child who has not gained and maintained his weight with the planned or unwitting complicity of his mother.

In conclusion, it has been suggested in this section that the high-risk population for obesity is influenced by age, sex, socioeconomic status, and ethnic and family characteristics. None of these factors is sufficient as a predictor of obesity, and predictions must be based upon an interaction of several factors. For example, while ethnic factors are surely of great importance, they cannot be viewed independently of national influences. In support of this viewpoint, Dr. Garn has noted:

> A Japanese from Tokyo or a Chinese from Taiwan, is still today far less fat than his American-born cousin in San Francisco or Chicago. After two generations in the U.S.A., Japanese-fat-thicknesses increase from below the 5th percentile to the U.S.A. 50th percentile or above.[52]

Therefore none of these factors is a singularly good predictor of obesity, and it follows that membership in one or more high-risk groups in no way sets a ceiling on the amount of change possible for any individual. Knowledge of the existence of the differential high risk for obesity associated with group membership would, however, serve as a guideline for means of adapting particular weight reduction programs to the needs of specified groups.

HOW DO PEOPLE BECOME OBESE?

It has been suggested that the literature pertaining to the causes of obesity abounds with hunches but hardly any controlled study to establish the facts.[53] This may be due in part to the proliferation of different types of obesity,[54] to the complexity of various mechanisms and responses relating to weight management, and to ethical constraints that properly limit the type of experimentation possible. While the range of facts may not be compelling, theories about the etiology of obesity abound. These

20

theories can be crudely divided among social, psychological, and biological explanations.

The strong association between socioeconomic, cultural, and familial factors seen in the research reviewed in the preceding section strongly supports the notion that social-psychological factors contribute to, if not cause, obesity. As will be seen in the following chapter, psychological explanations of obesity have not tended to be fruitful sources for hypotheses concerning the means through which obesity can be controlled. Beyond this limitation there has been little in the psychological literature to confirm the hunches common among laymen and professionals that the psychological make-up of obese persons distinguishes them as much from the nonobese population as does their size.

Drs. Moore, Stunkard, and Srole[55] extracted data from the Midtown Manhattan Study which did show that obese subjects had higher scores on three of nine measures − "immaturity," "rigidity," and "suspiciousness." While immaturity might coincide with the popular lay and psychiatric [56] notion that obese persons are self-indulgent, the rigidity finding would tend to contradict this and the finding concerning suspiciousness is essentially irrelevant. Furthermore, other researchers have adduced data showing that psychological adjustment is not closely related to obesity. For example, Silverstone,[57] working with the highly touted Cornell Medical Index, found that obesity and psychological health were actually inversely related in 344 Londoners of both sexes. He showed that 10 percent of the normal-weight men and 40 percent of the normal-weight women presented profiles indicating disturbance in contrast to 7 and 33 percent respectively of the markedly obese men and women. A facetious commentator might suggest that the very absence of psychological findings among obese persons is a pathognomonic sign of their disturbance in an apparent effort to sustain credence in an hypothesis despite contrary data. Even this assumption can be refuted, however, on the basis of treatment results to be reviewed in the next chapter which demonstrate that effective treatment is not associated with the manifestation of any discernible adverse psychological reaction.

While the social concomitants of obesity seem to be of importance, and the psychological concomitants seem to be of dubious value, biological explanations of obesity have considerable appeal. These explanations are legion, but only three will be mentioned here. The first is the role of genetics in the etiology of obesity. Genetic factors have been clearly shown to influence the occurrence of obesity in animals and, by analogy, the assumption has been made that obesity in humans is also subject to genetic transmission. While research with animals permits the experimental manipulation of breeding patterns, this is clearly not possible in humans. Therefore such data as are available are derived from what might be considered descriptive rather than experimental research — i.e., the observation of trends as they naturally occur rather than the controlled management of these trends. In one such study, several investigators[58] observed that less than 9 percent of the children of nonobese parents were obese, while obesity was found in 40 and 80 percent of the children born to one and two obese parents respectively. There are, however, a multitude of possible explanations for such an observation, not the least of which is the possible influence of parents who do or do not overeat. Moreover, while much is known about human genetics, Dr. Stanley Garn has noted that the precise means of transmission of genes relating to fattening and fleshing are not clearly understood.[59]

The second set of etiological hypotheses concerns the possibility that neuroanatomical aberrations may be the precursors of obesity, some of these affecting the experience of satiety and others affecting metabolic functioning. The experience of satiety requires the transmission of a highly complex set of signals within the body. Grossman described the process wherein satiety occurs in the following way:

> Food is metered in the mouth, pharynx and stomach. The nature of the detectors in these areas are not known, but volume appears to be of great importance and hence distension receptors can be postulated. When the signals to the brain from these detectors reach a certain level feeding reflexes are inhibited; eating ceases. The setting of this mechanism is probably determined by energy balance. This setting displays considerable inertia; the volume of food ingested tends to remain constant and only changes slowly in response to positive or negative energy loads. How the energy loads influence the setting, how the tissues tell the brain how much energy they have stored, is unknown.[60]

While the nuances of the process may not be known, it is believed that as many as three fourths of the obese population may not ever experience either hunger or satiety,[61] or if they do experience hunger it may not be in association with the same inner cues which trigger hunger responses in nonobese persons.[62]

The metabolic factors which are believed to play a role in the etiology of obesity can have varied origins, some of which are attributable to hypothalamic and cortical dysfunctions. It is doubtful, however, that metabolic disturbances are the prime causes of obesity and they may, in fact, only be secondarily reactive to the occurrence of obesity. The minor role of metabolic factors in obesity has been pointed out by Dr. Gilbert B. Forbes of the University of Rochester School of Medicine with his observation that when obese people add weight:

> ... most of the excess weight is fat, for in reality this is the only organ in the body capable of such great expansion in size and of

storing the excess energy. Patients lose weight in predictable fashion on starvation or controlled low calorie diets, and urinary nitrogen loss is in the expected direction. These facts alone speak strongly against a metabolic cause.[63]

The third factor associated with the onset of obesity is the recently discovered histological observation concerning the cell count in obese persons. Recent research in rats[64] and in humans,[65] for example, have shown that there is little change in the number of adipose cells comprising an individual's "fat pads" following a given point in infant development. When obesity occurs following the completion of this developmental phase, it results in an expansion in the size of adipose cells rather than the number of these cells. The same investigators have shown that enlarged cells are curiously less responsive to insulin than cells of normal size and, as insulin would aid the metabolism (conversion into energy) of carbohydrates (starches and sugars), people with a high percentage of enlarged cells would be expected to suffer from an inability to efficiently metabolize carbohydrates, a fact which would complicate treatment.

After reviewing the varied explanations of obesity, Mayer[66] and others[67] concluded that whatever the predisposing factors, virtually all obesities have in common an association between an excessive caloric intake and a deficient level of energy expenditure. Over forty years ago, Newburgh and Johnston arrived at a similar conclusion, noting that cases of obesity are:

> . . . never directly caused by abnormal metabolism but are always due to food habits not adjusted to the metabolic requirement — either the ingestion of more food than is normally needed or the failure to reduce the intake in response to a lowered requirement.[68]

Obesity, then, whatever its root causes, is seen as the result of a positive energy balance. When the energy balance can be reversed, obesity can be overcome. It is this model of obesity which serves the basis of the intervention plan which will be outlined shortly.

WHAT CAN BE DONE ABOUT OBESITY?

General Considerations. Thus far it has been asserted that obesity is a common problem which may have already reached epidemiological proportions in America, which has a differential probability of occurring among different groups within the society, which has an uncertain origin, and which is associated almost invariably with a positive energy balance. Of the some 2,000 lay and professional papers that have been published about obesity within the past quarter century alone, many are addressed to treatment. And of these, some are frankly fraudulent efforts to enrich their promoters[69] while others are well-intended professional efforts which have produced, with not many exceptions, mediocre results. For example, one authoritative group concluded that:

> ... most obese patients will not remain in treatment. Of those who do remain in treatment, most will not lose significant poundage, and of those who do lose weight, most will regain it promptly.[70]

This dismal conclusion must suppress the enthusiasm of anyone who would contemplate entering treatment for obesity. While it is essential that he ascertain that he is free of contraindications to weight loss — "diverticulitis, gout and tuberculosis are examples of diseases commonly considered as having contraindications to weight reduction"[71] — and that he consult his physician prior to embarking upon a weight reduction program, he can improve the probability of a successful outcome if he chooses a program with four major characteristics.

First it is essential that the program be comparatively free of side effects. Some drug and surgical procedures may cause more harm than good. For example, the Public Health Service[72] has shown that the use of diuretics has little effectiveness in the treatment of obesity and may result in serious renal damage. Furthermore, the use of appetite-depressing drugs related to amphetamines may be effective for approximately six weeks but may be associated with many unpleasant side effects such as excessive tension and gastrointestinal distress, as well as creating serious additional risks for persons suffering from cardiac diseases.

An equally serious menace, however, is found in programs which produce short-range weight changes. Short-range weight loss is gratifying to the woman wishing to shape up to wear a bikini or to the man who wishes to wear his college prom tuxedo to his daughter's wedding. Furthermore, the weight-conscious adults of this nation are likely to embark on what often becomes a series of short-range diets. Commenting on this, Wyden stated:

> The average American "diet" has been charted to last between sixty and ninety days, but the dieter is off the diet during rougly half the time. He goes on 1.25 diets a year .... Dieting is a seasonal endeavor. Sales of diet products climb in January and February, when dieters suffer post-Christmas guilt, and in May and June, when they strain to attain respectable bathing suit figures. Sales sag sharply in October and reach a 35 per-cent-below-average depth in December.[73]

The problem associated with such a pattern is that it may be associated with accretion of serum cholesterol in the cardiovascular system. In this connection, the Public Health Service forewarned:

> Serum cholesterol levels are elevated during periods of weight gain, thus increasing the risk of deposition. There is no evidence to show that once cholesterol is deposited it can be removed by weight

reduction. It is possible that a patient whose weight has fluctuated up and down a number of times has been subjected to more atherogenic stress than a patient with stable though excessive weight.[74]

Therefore it seems as essential to make certain that the weight reduction program lead to a stable weight loss over time — a loss that can be maintained continuously — as it is essential to minimize the aversive side effects of any technique utilized in the service of weight reduction.

Any treatment which is dependent upon elaborate external supports, whether in the form of continuous professional contacts or extraordinary rituals, is unlikely to fulfill this requirement of maintained weight reduction. Therefore a second requirement of a suitable program is that it be maximally adapted to the supports of appropriate weight management available in the natural environment. In support of this viewpoint, Drs. Sydnor Penick and Albert Stunkard reached the following conclusion after reviewing evidence associating obesity with various environmental factors (among others):

> The traditional medical model could well be considered an inappropriate use of these findings. This model defines an authoritarian role for the physician, who prescribes a diet and appetite-depressing medication. The patient loses weight, if at all, in large part to please the doctor and to meet his expectations. When the relationship is terminated or attenuated, the patient discontinues the diet and regains weight.[75]

In the judgment of Penick and Stunkard, then, it is essential for the physician to extend his influence from mere relationship-based instigations of the patient to diet and take pills to the development of a behavioral change effort which permeates the important food- and eating-related environmental forces. It follows from this that an effective strategy for the treatment of obesity must develop an assortment of therapeutic actions which are likely to be replicated in the natural environment — home, office, elsewhere — over time, and it is suggested that education is the technique most likely to meet with success in this vein.

The third element of effective treatment, then, is the use of educational techniques, some of which are targeted to the obese person and some of which are targeted to significant people in his immediate environment. Educational techniques have the advantage of building skills for the management of varied situations, and of extending the effect of the intervention to other individuals as well. Thus, for example, when an obese mother is trained in the appropriate selection and management of food, the realized or potential obesity of others in the family may be curbed as well. In this way, education can serve a preventive function, prevention possibly being the only effective strategy in efforts to stem the tide of obesity.

The final requirement of an effective program for the control of obesity is more philosophical than it is practical: It is that the onus for weight gain and reduction must be appropriately placed upon the environment rather than upon the overweight person. Mayer has commented that, unlike most human afflictions, obesity is still considered to be a form of moral deviance for which the individual rather than his pathogenic environment is held responsible. [76] He asserted:

> The old view of medicine, that patients are sick because of their sins, including their lack of self-restraint — a view which has been generally abandoned in the Western world even in the matter of alcoholism — still dominates as far as obesity is concerned. Obesity, almost alone among all the pathologic conditions, remains a moral issue. [77]

Mayer's assertion has been borne out by several lines of investigation. The Maddox, Anderson, and Bogdonoff study[78] cited earlier reported that nonobese persons blame obese individuals as being responsible for their problem while persons with a broad array of other problems are not viewed as having this responsibility. Maddox and Liederman[79] later presented data suggestive of the fact that these same attitudes are often shared by professional persons charged with the care of obese individuals, and Maddox, Back, and Liederman[80] showed that the same attitudes even permeated the evaluations of obese persons themselves. Finally, working with a sample of obese adolescents, Canning and Mayer[81] showed that school counsellors were less apt to write reference letters for obese students than for nonobese students and that, as might be expected, the former group was less likely than the latter group to be accepted into colleges, despite the fact that their intelligence and achievement scores were not inferior to the scores of their normal-weight counterparts. [82] These and other investigations[83] show that obese adolescents and adults are generally victimized as much by the secondary social consequences of obesity — e.g., rejection and isolation from opportunities to have social experiences which would allow them to transcend their obesity — as by the primary implications of obesity itself. So great is this problem that it has been shown to adversely affect the very efforts designed to conquer obesity. For example, Drs. Goldblatt, Moore, and Stunkard asserted:

> It seems quite possible that the lack of success in the control and treatment of obesity stems from the fact that until now physicians have thought of obesity as always being abnormal. This is certainly not true for persons in the lower socioeconomic population. Obesity may always be unhealthy, but it is not always abnormal. [84]

There is perhaps a reciprocal interaction between the concepts of obesity as deviance and the view that psychological forces underlie the problem of obesity. Some time ago, Drs. Moore, Stunkard, and Srole[85] reached the conclusion that the preoccupation with obesity as a psychological problem may have resulted from the fact that physicians were more apt to be asked to treat rich patients than poor patients, the environmental precipitators of obesity being more evident in the latter group. In fact, Szasz has expressed the view that Freud's conception of neurosis was similarly in error due to a bias in his observations, which were restricted to upper-class female patients.[86] In any case, it seems safe to conclude that the moralization found to surround obesity is responsible for creating a counterproductive element in treatment which may be a direct consequence of the psychologizing about obesity.

In summary, it can be said that an effective intervention program addressed to the control of obesity should minimize unwanted side effects by, for example, leading to a maintainable loss of weight, should rely as much as possible upon those controls of behaviors related to weight management which are found in the natural environment, should use educationally oriented techniques, and should avoid stigmatizing the obese person as being morally inferior. Beyond these requirements, it is of course essential that the treatment be scientifically based, that it have limited and known side effects, that it have fairly widespread appeal or at least that its efficacy be known for specific populations, and above all that it be effective.

Specific Proposals. This book will describe in detail a three-pronged approach to the management of obesity. The three targets of the approach are management of the environment related to eating and exercise, direct manipulation of eating through nutritional management, and direct manipulation of the amount of energy expenditure through enhancement of the probability of an appropriate increase in exercise.

Situational management. The situational approach to the control of obesity proceeds from a recognition of the relative importance of the environmental forces which shape the character of the eating and energy expenditure behaviors related to obesity. More than this, however, it also specially eschews any effort to attribute either the occurrence of obesity or the failure of efforts to curb obesity to any forces other than those which are identifiable in the environment. This approach, then, should be viewed in sharp contrast to others which start from an assumption that forces within the individual either initiate or sustain problematic patterns of behavior.

When behavior conforms to the simplistic predictions — e.g., as when an obese man indulges in overeating — observers would agree that his behavior is under environmental control. However, when behavior appears to contradict these predictions — as when an obese man refuses or only

27

gingerly nibbles at proffered sweets — the mettle of the observer is tested. On these occasions the concept of "Inner Man" is likely to be evoked as a mediating construct linking stimulus (cake) and response (eating) to explain an apparent change in the normal function of the stimulus. Dr. B.F. Skinner has written pointedly about the conditions associated with and the futility resulting from application of the concept of Inner Man in the following words:

> ... the Inner Man is most often invoked when the behavior to be explained is unusual, fragmentary, or beyond control — unusual with respect to other parts of a man's behavior, fragmentary with respect to his behavior as a whole, and beyond the control of the rest of him as a person. But the "rest of him" must also be explained, and when all parts have been assembled, the Inner Man behaves very much like the Outer. Nothing has been gained by this animistic practice but the Inner Man still calls for explanation. Indeed, we now face our original problems in a much more difficult form. It is surprising that psychologists permit their task to be set forth in this troublesome way.[87]

For Skinner, then, Inner Man notions such as "self-control" and "guilt" are seen to add little to either the explanation or control of behavior. In fact they may actually be viewed as factors which reduce the likelihood of behavior control activities insofar as they introduce irrelevancies into such efforts or insofar as they permit the rationalization of failures.

The same events which are explained by reference to terms such as "self-control" can be explained more fruitfully in the language of situational control. For example, the obese man who refuses a piece of his favorite pastry might, to the hurried observer, seem to be acting in a manner contrary to the obvious environmental influence. But the more patient observer who views his actions over time might see that the refusal of the pastry set the occasion for the man to later tell his wife of his virtue. He might then receive from her the just desserts of his action — rewards far more valuable to him than a piece of cake. What is being claimed here, then, is that the man who forebears is not more virtuous than he who indulges; rather he more wisely defers an immediate pleasure for one of greater value which is his later. Whether he takes his immediate reward and eats it or defers to a subsequent reward, therefore, he is seen to be not under "self-control" but under the control of the environment which actually plays two roles: It creates the conditions in which a choice is made necessary — creates temptation if you will — and it does or does not strengthen the likelihood that forebearance will take place. Some of these events are under the primary control of the obese person while others are under the control of significant persons with whom he interacts. Therefore the range of situations with which the interventionist must be concerned are few but complex and may be summarized in the following diagram:

		Primarily Controlled by Subject	Primarily Controlled by Others
To Be Increased	Events that set the occasion for desirable behavior	A	B
	Events that follow and strengthen desirable behavior		
To Be Decreased	Events that set the occasion for problematic behavior	C	D
	Events that follow and strengthen problematic behavior		

In using this format it should be clear that the entries in each cell will differ for each individual owing to personal idiosyncrasy and to differences in his social situation. For example, there has been considerable evidence that shows that obese persons eat at less regular intervals and less in association with conventional mealtimes than persons of normal weight. This supposition that obese persons may eat less regularly than normal-weight persons was confirmed in another investigation[88] which revealed that obese subjects were more likely to skip breakfast entirely, miss lunch occasionally, and vary widely in dinner hour, particularly on weekends, when contrasted with nonobese persons. This variability in eating patterns will be shown to be problematic for overeaters whose behavior with respect to food thereby is allowed to occur in many places so that those places may become learned cues for problematic eating. The occasion of fixed mealtimes and support for eating at least three focal meals daily will be shown to be essential elements in the management of problem eaters. A single man who takes his own meals may exercise control of this schedule, and therefore this aspect of his environment would fall within cell A of the diagram. Conversely, for a married man whose wife schedules mealtimes, the appropriate cell entry would be B. However, if the single man worked at an occupation for which mealtimes were more under the influence of variable job routines than under the control of his nutritional needs, the appropriate cell entry would be C, while the D cell entry would be used for a man whose wife was also a problematic eater who scheduled meals at irregular intervals and consisting of varying amounts of nourishment. Categorized in this manner, the situational events related to eating may be seen to fall within one of two major intervention systems — one oriented to increasing or strengthening appropriate cues and one oriented to decreasing or weakening inappropriate cues—each of which will be shown to suggest specific intervention techniques.

Nutrition management. The second element of the intervention program recommended here is the management of food selection and preparation. Most responsible programs aimed at weight control contain some reference to weight reduction. Unfortunately these programs often take on the quality of "get thin quick" schemes. Some of the least responsible diet management programs involve the selection of one or more of a small number of foods characterized as nutritional marvels for the would-be dieter. Cabbage, rice, eggs, steak, fish, fruit, and milk, among a great many others, have been suggested as single-food diets promising startling effectiveness. Under the best of circumstances, however, these diets lead to only a temporary loss of weight, as weight is regained following a return to a normal diet. Fasting is another dietary manipulation which has been used effectively in extreme situations such as those requiring pre-surgical rapid weight loss but, like fad-food diets, fasting is associated with a rapid weight gain following the termination of the fast. In one study,[89] for example, 25 patients hospitalized for a medically supervised fast lost an average of just under 30 pounds in 24 days. Within six months of discharge from the ward, however, their average weight was two pounds greater than their pre-fasting weight. The third type of approach leading to time-limited loss is the use of dietary aids such as formula diets, low-calorie sweeteners (e.g., saccharin), and low-calorie bulk (e.g., methyl cellulose). As with fad diets and fasting, however, these unnatural dietary limits prove effective for a short duration, if at all. In view of these facts, it is now generally recognized that more temperate approaches are to be preferred.

Rather than relying upon eccentric foods, fasting, or dietary aids, it is generally recognized that education in sound dietary practice is an essential in durable weight control programs. In fact the Public Health Service has asserted that "education of the patient . . . is imperative."[90] The effects of dietary education have been clearly shown in a recent study of the interrelationship between the nutrition knowledge of mothers and the manner in which they fed their families.[91] The study revealed that mothers with the lowest level of nutritional knowledge tended not only to feed their families foods with the least nutrient value but also to be overly permissive and to train their children in the least beneficial eating habits.

Beyond general agreement among experts that nutrition education is essential, there is also agreement that minimal diets for men and women should be 1,500 and 1,000 calories respectively.[92] In a recent study which carefully monitored the food intake of dieting adults, for example, successful dieters consumed 1,511 calories and 68 percent of their minimum daily food requirements, while unsuccessful dieters averaged 1,748 calories per day.[93] The margin of difference between effective and ineffective diets, therefore, can be found for some people to be as little as a single rich dessert. While there is some fairly strong evidence that the diet should be carefully controlled with respect to its effect upon the cholesterol level within the body (due to a strong association between cholesterol, obesity, and cardiac illness),[94] it appears as though the best diet for weight reduction is balanced with respect to the essential nutrients. In fact, contrary to a popular misconception, research over the years[95] has tended to show that balanced diets are not only as conducive to weight loss as diets weighted toward high fat or high protein, but in addition are more likely to be followed over time. Therefore the second element in the approach advocated by the present authors calls for the general nutritional reeducation of the weight loser toward the end of achieving a new set of balanced, calorie-restricted food choices.

Exercise. One of the unfortunate consequences of modern civilization is the high priority which it has placed upon the saving of labor. In 1962, there were 78 million registered motor vehicles in the United States, almost six for every ten persons over the age of 21. These cars were driven 713 billion miles and accounted for 85 percent of the travel within cities and 99 percent of rural travel.[96] With these resources, transportation rarely required energy expenditure. In addition, three out of every four homes had convenience appliances ranging from washing machines and dryers to almost automatic central dust-controlled units, and automation has reduced much of the exertion in industry. Each of these devices conspires to lower energy output. As the amount of energy consumed through exercise falls, food intake should be reduced in like amount. Regrettably this adjustment of consumption in coordination with reduced energy needs is infrequently made. This has led Mayer to the conclusion that "inactivity is the most important factor explaining the frequency of 'creeping' overweight in modern societies."[97]

There are three avenues toward the control of a positive energy balance: sharply reduce the consumption of energy as food; sharply increase the expenditure of energy as exercise; or moderately decrease food intake while moderately increasing energy output. In keeping with the general position being taken here, the third alternative would appear to offer the greatest promise of producing a maintainable long-term effect.

People vary greatly in the rate at which they expend energy through exercise. Researchers at the University of Michigan[98] have shown that there are statistically significant differences in the average amount of energy expended by blue- and white-collar workers between the ages of 30 to 59, with professional, managerial, sales, and clerical workers expending less energy than skilled and unskilled labor and service personnel. The same study also revealed, however, that managerial workers are more likely to engage in leisure-time activities which require heavy energy expenditure.

Other differences have been noted between the energy expenditure patterns of individual women and of obese and nonobese women.[99] In the latter area, Dr. Margen has shown that obese housewives spend 70 percent of their time in light activities such as sleeping, sitting activities, and personal activities and 29 percent of their time in moderate activities including shopping, walking, and standing. The comparable figures for nonobese housewives are 65 and 34 percent, indicating that obese women exercise vigorously approximately one-sixth less than nonobese women. This finding is particularly important when coupled with Mayer's observation that when obese and nonobese individuals do the same task, the former expend more energy in its performance than the latter.[100] Therefore while energy expenditure patterns are somewhat individual, it can be said that obese people exercise less but benefit more from their exercise than do nonobese people.

The adjustments needed to have a corrective effect upon the energy balance are not necessarily large or inconveniencing. For example, Mayer estimates that if a 150-pound man spends one hour walking in place of sitting he will spend from 100 to 550 additional calories depending upon his walking speed.[101] In the same vein, a 200-pound man would spend approximately one third more calories in the same activity, despite the observed "training effect" which seems to enable obese individuals to economize somewhat in their energy expenditure.[102] When adjustments are made in energy balance, three important weight-related effects can be expected. First, weight loss can be expected as increases in food intake will rarely exceed the increases in energy expenditure.[103] Second, there is likely to be a decrease in the amount of food eaten during the early stages of an increase in exercise. For example, it has been shown that men engaging in sedentary work consumed an average of 3,400 calories per day while those in light and heavy work consumed 2,600 and 3,200 calories respectively.[104] Finally, it has been estimated by Ancel Keys that 98 percent of the weight lost through diet and exercise is likely to be fat while only 75 percent of the weight lost is fat when a diet-only program is followed.[105] Finally, there is also evidence that those who pursue more active lives will be more likely to have longer lives, that is, that "physical activity and coronary heart disease are inversely related."[106] For example, while factors such as the characteristics of men who initially choose occupations cannot be overlooked, coronary disease was 1.7 times more likely among South Dakota nonfarmers than farmers, twice as likely for railroad clerks as compared with section hands, and 40 percent greater for Californians engaged in sedentary as opposed to active labor.[107] Therefore, both for its importance in weight control and as a preventive health measure, exercise should be a part of any program addressed to the management of obesity.

Conclusion. The three-pronged attack upon obesity described here — involving the management of the situational controls of eating and the management of energy consumption and expenditure — is believed to fulfill the major requirements of a successful obesity intervention program. It is based upon the use of procedures that can be sustained over time, with a minimum of external support due to a reliance upon educational techniques which exonerate the obese person of much of the personal responsibility for his problematic behavior. Each pair of the next six chapters will provide the theory and practical recommendations associated with each of the three phases of the treatment just introduced.

FOOTNOTES

1. Christakis, G. Community programs for weight reduction: Experience of the Bureau of Nutrition, New York City. *Canadian Journal of Public Health*, 1967, *58*, 499-504.
2. Wyden, P. *The overweight society*. New York: William Morrow, 1965.
3. U.S. Public Health Service. *Obesity and health*. Washington, D.C.: U.S. Government Printing Office, undated.
4. Baird, I.M. Obesity in adults. In I.M. Baird and A.M. Howard (Eds.), *Obesity: Medical and scientific aspects*. Edinburgh: E. and S. Livingstone, 1969, P. 21.
5. Christakis, *op. cit.*
6. Dwyer, J.T. and Mayer, J. Potential dieters: Who are they? *Journal of the American Dietetic Association*, 1970, *56*, 510-514.
7. Wyden, *op. cit.*, p. 1.
8. MacLeod, R.B. Impact of diet on behavior. *American Journal of Clinical Nutrition*, 1957, *5*, 108.
9. Fee, J.M., Wilson, N.L., and Wilson, R.H.L. Obesity: A gross national product. In N.L. Wilson (Ed.), *Obesity*. Philadelphia: F.A. Davis, 1969. Pp. 243-244.
10. Durnin, J.V.G.A. and Passmore, R. *Energy, work and leisure*. London: Heinemann, Educational Books Ltd., 1967.
11. See, for example, Mayer, J. *Overweight*. Englewood Cliffs, N.J.: Prentice-Hall, 1968, Chapter 2; and Behnke, A.R. New concepts in height-weight relationships. In Wilson, *Obesity, op. cit.*
12. Seltzer, C.C. and Mayer, J. A simple criterion of obesity. *Postgraduate Medicine*, 1965, *38*, A101-A107.
13. U.S. Public Health Service. *Weight, height, and selected body dimensions of adults*. Washington, D.C.: U.S. Government Printing Office, 1965.
14. *Ibid.*, p. 19.
15. Karpinos, B.D. Height and weight of Selective Service registrants processed for military service during World War II. *Human Biology*, 1958, *30*, 292-321; and Karpinos, B.D. Current height and weight of youths of military age. *Human Biology*, 1961, *33*, 335-354.
16. U.S. Public Health Service, *Weight, height, op. cit.*, p. 21.
17. Metropolitan Life Insurance Company, New York. New weight standards for men and women. *Statistical Bulletin*, 1969, *40* (Whole No. 3).
18. Montegriffo, V.M.E. Height and weight of a United Kingdom adult population with a review of anthropometric literature. *Annals of Human Genetics*, 1968, *31*, 389-399.
19. U.S. Public Health Service, *Obesity and health, op. cit.*, p. 2.
20. Seltzer and Mayer, *op. cit.*

21. *Ibid.*, p. A103.
22. Matiegka, J. The testing of physical efficiency. *American Journal of Physical Anthropology*, 1921, *4*, 223-230.
23. Franzen, R. Physical measures of growth and nutrition. In *School Health Research Monographs, No. 2*. New York: American Child Health Association, 1929.
24. Mayer, *op. cit.*, pp. 31-32.
25. Seltzer and Mayer, *op. cit.*
26. Mayer, *op. cit.*, pp. 30-31.
27. Garn, S.M., Rosen, N.N., and McCann, M.B. Personal communication, 1971.
28. U.S. Public Health Service, *Weight, height, op. cit.*
29. U.S. Public Health Service. *Skinfolds, body girths, biacromial diameter, and selected anthropometric indices of adults*. Washington, D.C.: U.S. Government Printing Office, 1970.
30. U.S. Public Health Serivce, *Obesity and health, op. cit.*
31. Srole, L., Langer, T.S., Michael, S.T., Opler, M.K., and Rennie, T.A.C. *Mental health in the metropolis: Midtown Manhattan study*. New York: McGraw-Hill, 1962.
32. Goldblatt, P.B., Moore, M.E., and Stunkard, A.J. Social factors in obesity. *Journal of the American Medical Association*, 1965, *192*, 97-102.
33. *Ibid.*, p. 100.
34. Dwyer and Mayer, *op. cit.*
35. Wyden, *op. cit.*
36. Goldblatt, Moore, and Stunkard, *op. cit.*
37. Maddox, G.L., Anderson, C.F., and Bogdonoff, M.D. Overweight as a problem of medical management in a public outpatient clinic. *American Journal of Medical Science*, 1966, *252*, 394-403.
38. Goldblatt, Moore, and Stunkard, *op. cit.*, p. 98.
39. Brown, I.C. *Understanding other cultures*. Englewood Cliffs, N.J.: Prentice-Hall, 1963. P. 22.
40. Titiev, M. *The science of man: An introduction to anthropology*. New York: Henry Holt, 1954. Pp. 351-352.
41. Cussler, M. and DeGive, M.L. *'Twixt the cup and the lip: Psychological and socio-cultural factors affecting food habits*. New York: Twayne Publishers, 1952. P. 38.
42. Lee, D. Cultural factors in dietary choice. *American Journal of Clinical Nutrition*, 1957, *5*, 167.
43. Dwyer, J.T., Feldman, J.J., and Mayer, J. The social psychology of dieting. *Journal of Health and Social Behavior*, 1970, *11*, 273-274.
44. Goldblatt, Moore, and Stunkard, *op. cit.*
45. Stunkard, A.J. Environment and obesity: Recent advances in our understanding of regulation of food intake in man. *Federation Proceedings*, 1968, *27*, 1367-1373.
46. Garn, S.M. Cultural and familial attitudes toward leanness and fatness. Paper presented at the meeting of the American Dietetic Association, Cleveland, October 1970.
47. Garn, S.M. and Pao, E.M. Nutritional problems and nutritional solutions in long-term studies of growth and aging. In Ohio Department of Health, Ohio Nutrition Committee. *A report on the 9th Conference on Human Nutrition: "Nutrition in a mod world."* Columbus: Ohio State University Press, 1968.
48. Garn, *op. cit.*
49. *Ibid.*
50. *Ibid.*, p. 5.
51. Garn, *op. cit.*
52. *Ibid.*, p. 3.
53. Cappon, D. Obesity. *Canadian Medical Association Journal*, 1958, *79*, 570.
54. U.S. Public Health Service, *Obesity and health, op. cit.*, p. 33.
55. Moore, M.E., Stunkard, A., and Srole, L. Obesity, social class, and mental illness. *Journal of the American Medical Association*, 1962, *181*, 962-966.
56. Bruch, H. *The importance of overweight*. New York: Norton, 1957.
57. Silverstone, J.T. Psychological factors in obesity. In Baird and Howard, *Obesity: Medical and scientific aspects, op. cit.*
58. Johnson, M.L., Burke, B.S., and Mayer, J. Relative importance of inactivity and overeating in the energy balance of obese high school girls. *American Journal of Clinical Nutrition*, 1956, *4*, 37-44.

59. Garn, S.M. The genetics of normal human growth. In L. Gedda (Ed.), *De Genetica Medica* (2nd International Conference of Human Genetics, Rome 1961). Rome: Gregor Mendel Institute, 1962.
60. Grossman, M.I. Satiety signals. *American Journal of Clinical Nutrition*, 1960, *8*, 565-566.
61. Hollifield, G., Owen, J.A., Lindsay, R.W., and Parson, W. Effects of prolonged fasting on subsequent food intake in obese humans. *Southern Medical Journal*, 1964, *57*, 1012-1016.
62. Stunkard, A.J. Obesity and the denial of hunger. *Psychosomatic Medicine*, 1959, *21*, 281-289.
63. Forbes, G.B. The great denial. *Nutrition Reviews*, 1967, *25*, 355.
64. Knittle, J.L. and Hirsch, J. Effect of early nutrition on the development of rat epididymal fat pads: Cellularity and metabolism. *Journal of Clinical Investigation*, 1968, *47*, 2091-2098.
65. Hirsch, J., Knittle, J.L., and Salans, L.B. Cell lipid content and cell number on obese and nonobese human adipose tissue. *Journal of Clinical Investigation*, 1966, *45*, 1023 (Abstract); and Salans, L.B., Knittle, J.L., and Hirsch, J. The role of adipose cell size and adipose tissue insulin sensitivity in the carbohydrate intolerance of human obesity. *Journal of Clinical Investigation*, 1968, *47*, 153-165.
66. Mayer, *op. cit.*
67. For example, Wilson, N.L., Farber, S.M., Kimbrough, L.D., and Wilson, R.H.L. Development and perpetuation of obesity: An overview. In Wilson, *Obesity, op. cit.*
68. Newburgh, L.H. and Johnston, M.W. The nature of obesity. *Journal of Clinical Investigation*, 1930, *8*, 197-213.
69. Wyden, *op. cit.*
70. Cornell Conferences on Therapy. The management of obesity. *New York State Journal of Medicine*, 1958, *58*, 87.
71. U.S. Public Health Service, *Obesity and health, op. cit.*, p. 71.
72. *Ibid.*, pp. 55-56. See also Modell, W. Status and prospect of drugs for overeating. *Journal of the American Medical Association*, 1960, *173*, 1131-1136.
73. Wyden, *op. cit.*, p. 8.
74. U.S. Public Health Service, *Obesity and health, op. cit.*, p. 71.
75. Penick, S.B. and Stunkard, A.J. Newer concepts of obesity. *Medical Clinics of North America*, 1970, *54*, 752.
76. Mayer, *op. cit.*
77. *Ibid.*, p. 1.
78. Maddox, Anderson, and Bogdonoff, *op. cit.*
79. Maddox, G.L. and Liederman, V. Overweight as a social disability with medical implications. *Journal of Medical Education*, 1969, *44*, 210-220.
80. Maddox, G.L., Back, K., and Liederman, V. Overweight as social deviance and disability. *Journal of Health and Social Behavior*, 1968, *9*, 287-298.
81. Canning, H. and Mayer, J. Obesity: Its possible effect on college acceptance. *New England Journal of Medicine*, 1966, *275*, 1172-1174.
82. Canning, H. and Mayer, J. Obesity: An influence on high school performance. *American Journal of Clinical Nutrition*, 1967, *20*, 352-354.
83. Dwyer, Feldman, and Mayer, *op. cit.*
84. Goldblatt, Moore, and Stunkard, *op. cit.*, p. 102.
85. Moore, Stunkard, and Srole, *op. cit.*
86. Szasz, T. *The myth of mental illness.* New York: Hoeber-Harper, 1967.
87. Skinner, B.F. *Contingencies of reinforcement: A theoretical analysis.* New York: Appleton-Century-Crofts, 1969. Pp. 272-273.
88. Schachter, S. and Gross, L.P. Manipulated time and eating behavior. *Journal of Personality and Social Psychology*, 1968, *10*, 98-106.
89. MacCuish, A.C. and Munro, J.F. Follow-up study of refractory obesity treated by fasting. *British Medical Journal*, 1968, *1*, 91-92.
90. U.S. Public Health Service, *Obesity and health, op. cit.*, p. 52.
91. Eppright, E.S., Fox, H.M., Fryer, B.A., Lamkin, G.H., and Vivian, V.M. Nutrition knowledge and attitudes of mothers. *Journal of Home Economics*, 1970, *62*, 327-332.
92. For example, see U.S. Public Health Service, *Obesity and health, op. cit.*
93. Howard, A.N. Dietary treatment of obesity. In Baird and Howard, *Obesity: Medical and scientific aspects, op. cit.*

94. Epstein, F.H. and Ostrander, L.D. Detection of individual susceptibility toward coronary disease. *Progress in Cardiovascular Diseases,* 1971, *13,* 324-342; and Montoye, H.J., Epstein, F.H. and Kjelsberg, M.O. Relationship between serum cholesterol and body fatness. *American Journal of Clinical Nutrition,* 1966, *18,* 397-406.

95. Brewer, W.D., Cederquist, D.C., Williams, B., Beegle, R.M., Dunsing, D., Kelley, A.L., and Ohlson, M.A. Weight reduction of law-fat and low-carbohydrate diets: II. Utilization of nitrogen and calcium. *Journal of the American Dietetic Association,* 1952, *28,* 213-217; and Fletcher, R.F., McArrick, Y., and Crooke, A.C. Reducing diets: Weight loss of patients on diets of different composition. *British Journal of Nutrition,* 1961, *15,* 53-58.

96. Urban America, Inc. *Our people and their cities: Chart book.* Washington, D.C.: Urban America, Inc., undated.

97. Mayer, *op. cit.* p. 82.

98. Cunningham, D.A., Montoye, H.J., Metzner, H.L., and Keller, J.B. Physical activity at work and active leisure as related to occupation. *Medicine and Science in Sports,* 1969, *1,* 165-170.

99. Margen, S. Energy balance with increasing weight. In Wilson, *Obesity, op. cit.*

100. Mayer, *op. cit.*

101. *Ibid.,* p. 71.

102. Cunningham, D.A. and Falkner, J.A. The effect of training on aerobic and anaerobic metabolism during a short exhaustive run. *Medicine and Science in Sports,* 1969, *1,* 65-69; Bray, G.A. Effect of caloric restriction on energy expenditure in obese patients. *The Lancet,* 1969, *192,* 397-398; and Bloom, W.L. and Eidex, M.F. The comparison of energy expenditure in the obese and lean. *Metabolism,* 1967, *16,* 685-692.

103. Buskirk, E.R. Increasing energy expenditure: The role of exercise. In Wilson, *Obesity, op. cit.*

104. Mayer, J., Roy, P., and Mitra, K.P. Relation between caloric intake, body weight and physical work: Studies in an industrial male population in West Bengal. *American Journal of Clinical Nutrition,* 1956, *4,* 169-175.

105. Keys, A. Body composition and its change with age and diet. In E.S. Eppright, P. Swanson, and C.A. Iverson (Eds.), *Weight control.* Ames: Iowa State College Press, 1955.

106. Epstein, F.H. The epidemiology of coronary heart disease: A review. *Journal of Chronic Diseases,* 1965, *18,* 765.

107. *Ibid.,* p. 766.

Chapter 2
THE BEHAVIORAL PSYCHOLOGY OF EATING

Most writers concerned with the general problem of obesity accept the notion that corpulence is the result of overeating, underexercising, or both. Two paths diverge from this essential agreement in efforts to explain why or how individuals happen to allow their energy balance equation to become so imbalanced as to permit bodily growth sometimes reaching three or four times the desirable level. One path seeks to explain *why* people overeat through reference to *psychological* mechanisms, while the other point of view seeks to explain *how* people come to behave in biologically inappropriate ways through reference to the *situational* controls of behavior. This chapter will discuss each of these approaches in turn in an effort to lay the theoretical basis for the behavioral control of the energy balance.

PSYCHOLOGICAL STUDIES

Two groups of studies subsume most of the writing concerned with the psychological aspects of overeating. The first approach attempts to use an essentially inferential means of categorizing those who overeat from those who use appropriate eating controls. In one such study, Mendelson suggests that a continuum with a range of degrees of disturbance may be the best manner in which to characterize obese patients.[1] At one end of the continuum are patients who are emotionally stable. In Mendelson's research, approximately one fifth of his sample are in this category. A second point on the continuum includes patients who eat to defend against emotional tensions of various kinds, patients for whom obesity poses no real problem. At the most severely disturbed end of the continuum are those patients for whom obesity is a central problem, patients for whom food and its consumption are major preoccupations. Analogues to Mendelson's continuum are found in Hamburger's classification of eating disturbances.[2] At the point of least disturbance are found people who overeat in response to emotional tensions, times of transitional stress. A little further along are those who eat as a substitute gratification for extended periods of time. A third group includes patients who overeat almost constantly as a means of warding off emotional upheaval, most commonly depression. Finally, patients who are addicted to food are found at the extremely pathological end of the continuum.

The second approach is derived from the postulates of the psychoanalytic writers. Dr. Hilde Bruch of the Baylor University School of Medicine, perhaps the most influential of these writers, speculated that obesity is a consequence of personality defects in which body size becomes the expressive organ of an underlying psychological conflict.[3] In other words, obesity is viewed as a symptom of a deep psychological conflict. The origin of this conflict is believed by Bruch and others to rest in the early life experiences of the individual. For example, Deri concludes her review of the subject with the conclusion that:

> The psychological interpretation of obesity can certainly not be separated from the question of orality and thus implies the whole psychoanalytic theory of the various stages of psychosexual development and the various developmental phases of object relationship.[4]

Some writers believe that obesity is a consequence of disturbances during the "anal" period, which is believed to be the time when the young child seeks to establish his independence while his parents seek vigorously to bring his bowel and bladder functions under social control. The character structure of the adult "fixated at" or preoccupied with the challenges of the anal state are believed by psychoanalytic writers to be concerned with orderliness or compulsivity, autonomy, and/or defenses against heterosexuality. They would therefore assert that overeating is a compulsive habit wherein the individual both manifests his defiance of those who would control his consumatory behavior while at the same time protecting him from heterosexual experiences by virtue of the invulnerability or unattractiveness offered by excess weight.

Modern psychoanalytically oriented writers have searched for an explanation of the maladaptive symptom — obesity — in the early life experience of the obese individual. For example, Hilde Bruch has sought the precursors of obesity in parent-child interactions with the following observations:

> The early feeding histories of many fat and anorexic patients have been reconstructed with great detail. Often they are conspicuous by their blandness. The parents feel that there is nothing to report: the child never gave any trouble, ate exactly what was put before him; the mother was the envy of her friends and neighbors because her child did not fuss about food, nor was he negativistic during the classic "period of resistance." This goodness was reported for other areas, too, like cleanliness, no rough play or destructive behavior, and no disobedience or back talking. Several mothers . . . would

report with pride how they always "anticipated" their child's needs, never permitting him to "feel hungry."[5]

One of the mechanisms through which parents may inadvertently induce their offspring to eventually become obese is believed by Dr. Bruch to be on the one hand an inappropriate use of food in response to various emotional stress signals by the child while on the other hand a failure to respond with the provision of food in response to hunger.[6] In this manner it is believed that eating can become a response to almost every strong emotion, a learned reaction which can lead to highly inappropriate food habits during adolescence and adulthood. Thus the writers with this orientation assert that the eating disturbances of obese persons (as well as those who severely undereat, known as "anorexic" persons) are frequently the result of lifelong patterns of pathogenic interaction between the individual and key figures in his environment.

Accepting the psychodynamic notions of personality development, numerous authors have sought to expand the dynamic viewpoint to include a classification of the various possible manifestations of these conflicts in adult life. Deri[7] classifies these psychoanalytic writings into three groups. The first is concerned with the unconscious associations to the meaning of food itself. Food is understood to symbolize a range of essences from "mother's love" and the "symbolic incorporation of the breast" to father's phallus and "an impregnating substance." The second group is concerned with the symbolic meaning of the acts of oral intake and digestion. The libidinous qualities of these acts are characterized by the term "alimentary orgasm," while the sadistic quality is inherent in the phrase "cannibalistic incorporation of the mother." The third group of writers is concerned with the symbolic meaning of increased body size which occurs as a consequence of overeating. Explanations of this phenomenon range from a rejection of femininity through the "unconscious act of being castrated as well as protection against the danger of castration" to obesity as a symbol of pregnancy. In another vein, Bychowski postulates that the obese patient attempts identification with parents and/or siblings, and this "double identification interferes with the development of normal feminine personality and produces a trend towards masculinization."[8]

Finally, going beyond Deri's categorization, Drs. Harold and Helen Kaplan offer a veritable bestiary of explanations of the psychological meaning of overeating ranging from its serving as a means of self-indulgence to a means of self-punishment, among many others.[9] In light of these and related writings, it is not surprising to find several authors exploring the psychodynamically motivated resistances to weight loss. For example, Simon speculated that obese persons would resist giving up eating which for them served as a "depressive equivalent" or a response which took the place of feelings of depression.[10] This notion had actually been developed more extensively nine years earlier by Conrad[11] who attributed resistance to dieting to an unwillingness of the obese person to decrease the usefulness of his oral mechanisms as a means of solving emotional problems, to rebelliousness and an interest in preserving independence, to guilt associated with going off diets, to difficulty in being self-assertive when problematic foods are proffered, to hesitance to give up eating as a primary source of pleasure, and to a lack of motivation associated with a fear of failure. Beyond these speculations, Conrad suggested that obese individuals may resist dieting in order not to lose weight, large body size being associated with health and a protection against illness; strength, power, and greatness; fears of change, losing love, maturity, or narcissistic injury; identification with a fat parent; symbolic representation of pregnancy; protection against sexual temptation; low self-esteem; and high-strength tendencies toward self-punishment.

Numerous efforts have been made to validate the psychodynamic point of view, apparently without success. One problem stems from the fact that, as Stunkard has observed, "it has not been possible to define psychological characteristics of obese patients which will consistently distinguish them from nonobese patients."[12] All of us, for example, have within us a tendency to be self-defeating at times, but none of us acts in a self-defeating manner at all times. While some investigators have sought to show that some of us behave with great consistency in almost any situation, others have clearly shown that this is not possible. Researchers such as Patterson and Bechtel at the Oregon Research Institute have suggested that rather than having our behavior characterized as a "trait" in the hope of predicting what we will do across situations, our actions can best be characterized as "states" which stress the effect of the contiguous environment upon our actions.[13] If we do tend to behave in accordance with the demand characteristics of specific environments, then it would not be fruitful to seek to identify generally present traits.

A second problem with the use of psychodynamic notions in explaining obesity is the fact that predictions derived from the theory have not been consistently borne out in research. For example, if the psychodynamic conception of underlying personality weakness is correct, then it would be unwise to seek to aid the obese person to lose weight before surmounting the underlying conflict against which obesity is a defense in the belief that obesity is a "symptom that serves an important function in a precarious life adjustment."[14] An effort was made to validate this supposition in one study of weight loss under experimental conditions (a 600-calorie per day liquid diet over a period of 16 to 20 weeks) by six people whose weights ranged from 213 to 407 pounds at the start of the program.[15] Using multiple means of assessment, the researchers in this study concluded that:

> Those behavioral aberrations which were evident during weight loss but did not persist following weight loss included hunger symptoms, hostility-aggression, concern with the alteration of body size and ego boundary permeability. Those which persisted following weight loss included anxiety symptoms, depressive symptoms, sexual psychopathology, food-oriented behavior, and overestimation of body size. These observations suggest that instead of weight reduction resulting in a normal behavioral-metabolic state for obese patients, it more likely results in an abnormal state similar to that of starved nonobese individuals.[16]

Because the observations which served as the basis of the conclusions of this study are often based upon inferences from behavior rather than being the objects of direct assessment, caution must be used in evaluating them. In fact, the conclusions of this research have been rather seriously challenged in other studies. For example, Shipman and Plesset[17] studied the psychological consequences of dieting for 70 consecutive referrals to the Nutrition Clinic of the University of Pittsburgh and 81 patients under the care of a private Pittsburgh general practitioner. They found that depression and anxiety *diminished* among those patients who succeeded in following the prescribed diet and eventually losing weight, returning only when and if weight gain reappeared. Much the same conclusion was reached in a study by Cauffman and Pauley[18] whose 26 patients lost an average of 20 percent of body weight through 1,000-calorie diets supplemented by the use of the drugs prochlorperazine and amphetamine. They found that "patients who lost more than one pound per week were found to have fewer symptoms of depression. They also tended to be less suspicious and less sensitive."[19] Furthermore, the patients who met with success in dieting also reported a reduced compulsion to eat.

It is possible that the depression associated with dieting observed by psychoanalytically oriented writers may be more attributable to the physiological effects of diminished food supply than to any innate psychological predispositions to depression. That is, when the supply of food is curtailed, the amount of free calories to maintain normal functioning is naturally curtailed as well, with the probable result that a behavioral depression (i.e., the nonoccurrence of habitual behaviors[20]) will occur. Beyond inactivity attributable to an absence of food-supplied energy, the overeater who accommodates to a calorie-restricted regimen permitting the consumption of only one fourth to one half of his normal food intake also is asked to give up eating as a high probability activity which in many instances serves to punctuate and maintain the even flow of the events of the day. Denied this behavioral support he is, in the language of Thomas Szasz,[21] "gameless" or faced with a vacuum of stimulation created by the relative diminution of the importance of eating and food in his life. This characteristically results in a temporary behavioral disorganization whether one is forced to give up food, a job, a friend, or any of the many behavioral supports upon which everyone depends. Furthermore, the same phenomenon is likely to greet the successful dieter who has learned to accommodate to the social world as an obese person, being the brunt of jokes, being cued to behavior in a jolly manner consistent with commonplace stereotypes, being less physically vigorous than most, and being treated as a comparative outsider in many activities. As he becomes thin, it is necessary for him to develop a new set of social responses, and while these are being developed he may undergo a transitional behavioral disorganization which might be incorrectly attributed to underlying psychological distress by clinical observers.

In short, it is suggested that many of the psychological problems believed to generate obesity and problems in weight loss can be more profitably understood as reactions to obesity and dieting. Viewed in this manner, they are far more amenable to control than they would be if postulated as basic underlying characterological mechanisms. This possibility was recognized many years ago by Otto Fenichel, one of the giants of the psychoanalytic movement, when he raised the following question:

> Whenever a connection between an organic symptom and a mental conflict is encountered the first question must be: has the conflict produced the symptom or the symptom the conflict? No doubt there is sometimes a vicious circle, symptom and conflict perpetuating each other. [22]

Added to the criticisms that it may be unrealistic to seek out personality variables which have a broad-spectrum generality, that at least some of the assumptions in the psychodynamic point of view may not actually be borne out, and the apparent circularity of some of the beliefs is the final possibility that they may not be necessary or even relevant to effective treatment. This possibility was recognized by one of the proponents of the psychodynamic viewpoint, Susan Deri, who upon reviewing the basic theory and presenting a detailed analysis of therapy with an obese adolescent girl suggested that "the types of interpretations here described were important factors in therapy but were by no means considered to be the main therapeutic agents." [23] In the interest of parsimony, therefore, it is appropriate to move on to consider an alternate procedure — the behavioral control of overeating.

BEHAVIORAL STUDIES

One of the assumptions underlying the psychological studies is the view that personality factors such as feelings, thoughts, and ideas precede and set the occasion for behaviors such as eating or declining sweets in much the same manner that food consumption precedes and sets the occasion for the various consequences of eating ranging from good to poor health and from pleasant to unpleasant social experience. This set of relationships can be symbolized as follows:

Personality ⟶ Behavior ⟶ Consequences

e.g., tension, low sense of self-esteem	e.g., selecting high calorie foods over more desirable foods	e.g., problematically high blood-sugar level and social ostracism

Given this formulation, it is appropriate to intervene at the root of the problem — the personality with all of its affective and cognitive implications — in order to set the occasion for a change in behavior. Regrettably, efforts to use this approach in the treatment of overeating have met with less success than had been hoped for. Stuart has reviewed elsewhere[24] some of the possible explanations for the disappointing results flowing from personality-oriented treatments, explanations which include the high degree of speculation necessary in formulating hypotheses to guide treatment, the tendency for psychologically oriented treatment to focus upon problematic rather than constructive behaviors, and the likelihood that such treatments will also place the individual on the "hot seat" as it were, seeking to hold him accountable for behaviors which might better be changed through modificaton of the social and physical environmental forces which lead to the problematic behavior. Indeed, research workers interested in the control of overeating have of late turned to the modification of the environment as a preferred approach to modification of the individual (see Chapter 3), with the result that most of the assumptions guiding the intervention are testable through observable data, the techniques are oriented toward strengthening acceptable behavior, and the treatment strategy is oriented toward changing the responsible environment rather than compounding the guilt and shame of the overeater.

The model which underlies the behavioral approach to the study and treatment of overeating utilizes the same basic elements as the psychological model, but the point of entry is different. For the behavior analyst, the model can be represented symbolically as follows:

Behavior ⟶ Consequences ⟶ Thoughts; Feelings

e.g., underexercising through double parking in front of a store	e.g., weight gain with resulting loss of mobility	e.g., a sense of low self-esteem and depression

In this approach, it is not necessary to isolate and remediate forces deep in the psychological make-up of the individual in order to change his eating patterns. Instead, an effort is made to change his eating patterns so that he can have different experiences in the world, these experiences leading in turn to changes in the thoughts and feelings which comprise the messages which he gives himself. Because the changes in experience — e.g., greater mobility leading to greater social acceptance — are often delayed for some time because of the need to lose considerable amounts of weight, it is necessary to base the treatment upon a series of changes in the immediate environment which will make problem eating less probable so that the overeater is not faced with the impossible burden of giving up his pleasure in eating while having to wait weeks, months, or years before he finds alternative satisfactions. This section will review some of the studies which give rise to the notion that overeating behavior is under situational control; at the same time means of coping with the strong tendency toward overeating will be suggested. Among the situationally controlling variables which have received attention are the perception of time as a cue for eating, the availability of food, and the taste of food.

Early observations. In the development of ideas it is always difficult to identify a point of departure for a major trend of thought. Among those studying the situational control of overeating, however, the work of Stunkard[25] stands out as a monument. Working at the University of Pennsylvania, Dr. Stunkard devised an ingenious method for studying the responses of obese and nonobese adults. He arranged for each person to enter a laboratory setting at 9 a.m. following an overnight fast. Each volunteer was asked to swallow a gastric ballon attached to a Levin tube which was, in turn, attached to a kymograph. The ballon was inflated with 15 cm. of water and withdrawn until reaching the cardia, and the tube was then anchored at the nose with adhesive tape. For a four-hour period, subjects were asked at fifteen-minute intervals to report whether or not they were hungry. Some of these reports were associated with a kymographic tracing which indicated gastric contraction while other reports were not associated with what might be termed "hunger contractions." Fortunately for the purposes of this research, the tracings of the two groups were as sharply differentiated as the following two lines.

Gastric Motility

Absence of Gastric Motility

When the results of the obese and nonobese subjects were compared, it was shown that the nonobese individuals were significantly more likely than the obese individuals to report hunger in association with gastric motility. In light of these findings, Dr. Stunkard concluded that the cues for hunger are different for obese and nonobese persons. The critical question which this research posed was: If obese persons do not (while nonobese persons do) experience hunger in association with the obvious internal sensation of gastric contractions, what are the cues for eating for the obese?

Perceived time. One of the first investigators to seek an answer to this question was Dr. Stanley Schachter of Columbia University. Dr. Schachter undertook a series of studies, beginning in 1967, which was to win for him the Distinguished Scientists Award of the American Psychological Association and lay the groundwork for breakthroughs in the control of overeating. In one of these studies, undertaken by Dr. Schachter in collaboration with Dr. Larry P. Gross,[26] the responses of 22 Columbia undergraduates whose average weight was 31.5 percent above the norm were compared with the responses of 24 others from the same university whose average weight was only 2.6 percent above the norm. Volunteers in both groups who had eaten neither dinner nor large snacks during the one hour prior to the experiment were ushered into an experimental room where they were told, in a study beginning uniformly at 5:00 p.m., that they were to take part in a study of "the relation between physiological reactions and psychological characteristics, which required base level measurements of heart rate and sweat gland activity."[27] The experimenter then asked the subject to remove his wrist watch so that electrodes could be placed on his wrist and then left the subject alone in the room with two stimuli: a polygraph presumably recording his heart rate and galvanic skin responses and a clock. For one half of the subjects (half each of the obese and nonobese group), the clock was rigged to run at a rate which over 50 minutes would be 15 minutes slow while for the remaining subjects it was set to run 30 minutes fast. Thus while both groups began the experiment at 5:00 p.m., one group finished this phase of the study at what they believed was 5:35 p.m. while the other believed the time to be 6:20 p.m. – the actual time being 5:50 p.m. The experimenter then returned with a box of "Wheat Thins" which he began to eat, offering some to the subjects, and asked the subjects to complete an irrelevant pencil and paper task. The data for testing the principal hypothesis of the study—the belief that obese subjects would be more influenced by perceived time than nonobese subjects—were the number of crackers eaten. The data strongly supported the hypothesis, showing that obese subjects in the slow time condition ate 19.9 grams of crackers as opposed to the 37.6 grams eaten by obese subjects in the fast time condition, just the reverse of the results for nonobese subjects who ate 41.5 grams during the slow time condition and 16.0 grams during the fast time condition. These results appeared to show that the obese subject who thought that it was not yet time to be hungry ate less than those who thought it was time to eat, while nonobese subjects ate fewer crackers when they believed their dinner hour to have arrived or passed. To further test this conclusion, Drs. Schachter and Gross asked the obese subjects when they would normally eat dinner and found that there was a very strong relationship in the findings between the number of crackers eaten and the subject's belief that his dinner hour had or had not yet passed.

In an interesting footnote to this study, incidental data collected by Nisbett,[28] in a study to be discussed more fully below, indicated that while underweight and normal-weight subjects reported hunger to be a function of the length of time since their last meal (r=.30 and .28, respectively), there was literally no association (r=.00) between food deprivation and the report of hunger by obese persons. This would seem to add further support to the belief that environmental forces play a key role in conditioning the feeling of hunger by the obese.

Another study can be cited in the further development of this thesis. Working with two collaborators, Drs. Ronald Goldman and Melvin Jaffa, Dr. Schachter conducted a study which came to similar conclusions with the use of naturalistic data,[29] a conclusion invulnerable to some of the threats to validity inherent in elaborate experimental manipulations. This study involved interviews with 236 Air France flight personnel assigned to transatlantic routes. The flights left Paris at around noon, typically required seven to eight hours of flight time and landed in the Eastern Standard Time Zone at between 2:00 and 3:00 p.m. Crews usually ate one meal while on board, arriving at their destinations some time after their last meal but between the normal mealtimes at their points of disembarkation. When the interviews of the 101 overweight subjects were compared with those of the 135 normal-weight subjects, it was found that only 11.9 percent of the overweight as opposed to 25.3 percent of the normal-weight subjects had reported hunger. Therefore this study also indicates that the hunger of obese subjects is influenced by actual or perceived time rather than by more logical internal cues.

Food cues. Time may be a more strongly learned cue for feeling hungry for obese individuals as opposed to those who are not overweight. But associated with time are likely to be other cues for eating such as the availability or fragrance of food and the sight of others eating. In the same

46

study in which they investigated the relationship between time and hunger experienced by Air France personnel, Goldman, Jaffa, and Schachter[30] also reviewed the effect of food cues upon the eating of Jewish students (defined as those who attended a synagogue at least once during the foregoing year) at Columbia University on Yom Kippur. In the Jewish faith, Yom Kippur is the Day of Atonement for one's faults and a day of prayer for the dead. As a sign of atonement, Jews are expected to fast for 24 hours. During this fasting period it is probable that the cues for eating — i.e., the availability of food and the sight of others eating — are not very obvious if they are present at all. Accordingly it can be expected that obese Jews are more likely to go without eating than nonobese Jews. The results of this naturalistic observational study confirm the predictions, showing 83.3 percent of the obese Jewish students to have fasted as opposed to 68.8 percent of the nonobese Jews, a difference which could occur by chance only five times out of a hundred. If the results of this study can be generalized, then the stereotype about the obese person thinking constantly about food would have to be set aside or at least qualified to imply that the obese person is more likely than his more slender counterpart to think about food when food cues are present but less likely to do so in the absence of food cues. Before traditional beliefs can be set aside, however, more evidence is needed.

One source of the needed data is found in studies by Ross[31] and Johnson[32] of the eating behavior of obese and nonobese individuals when food is highly visible. Each study manipulated the visibility of food, through controlling the amount of illumination in which it could be viewed or through wrapping the food in transparent rather than nontransparent paper, and each study experimentally validated the supposition that the visibility of food is a greater influence upon the behavior of obese as opposed to nonobese persons.

Another study which demonstrates the notion that obese persons are more subject to the influence of food cues than nonobese persons was conducted by Nisbett.[33] Following the experimental design utilized by Schachter, Nisbett deceived his subjects into believing that they were participating in a study of psychophysiological responses. Following a brief period of interaction with a meaningless but nonetheless impressive procedure, subjects were then led into a second room where they were asked to fill out some questionnaires which they believed to be related to the psychophysiological investigation. In the room they found either one or three roast beef sandwiches and a bottle of soda. They were told that since they had to miss lunch in order to participate in the research they were entitled to eat as many sandwiches as they wished, being able to take additional sandwiches from the refrigerator at will. When left alone, overweight subjects were found to eat more sandwiches than normal subjects (2.32 as opposed to 1.88 sandwiches) when three sandwiches were in view; when only one sandwich was in view, however, overweight subjects ate less than the normal subjects (1.48 as opposed to 1.96 sandwiches).

Taken together, these studies would appear to vindicate the obese person from the accusation that he is obsessed with food, insofar as his eating is at least under situational control. But one may ask further for an explanation of how this preponderant amount of environmental influence might come about. At least a partial answer is found in the study of the effect of increasing difficulty (response cost) upon the eating behavior of obese and normal subjects.

Response cost. One unflattering explanation of why obese people may be more dependent upon the visual cues of food than are nonobese persons is that persons in the former group may be less willing to expend effort to secure food than persons in the latter. Working with Dr. Lucy Friedman, Dr. Stanley Schachter[34] asked subjects to fill out questionnaires while sitting at a littered desk. One of the items on the desk was a bag of almonds. For one half of the subjects the almonds were shelled while for the other half of the group, the almonds were not shelled. Of normal subjects in each condition, only one ate nuts which required shelling while 11 of 20 ate nuts which they did not have to shell. Of the 20 obese subjects in each condition, only one ate nuts which required shelling while 19 ate nuts which were already shelled. While it may be possible to explain the results by inferring that obese persons were less likely to wish to undergo the conspicuousness of eating nuts which required shelling, it is probably more parsimonious to conclude that the work required deterred the obese group from indulging.

Again displaying his genius for finding naturalistic means of collecting data, Dr. Schachter (along with Drs. Friedman and Handler) devised another means of testing the same phenomenon.[35] They did this by observing in Chinese and Japanese restaurants Occidental patrons who ate with chopsticks. It is clearly more cumbersome for a Westerner to use chopsticks in place of conventional silverware, particularly when the cuisine is oriental for it almost invariably is served in small morsels. It is therefore not surprising that over four times as many of the users of chopsticks (22.4 percent as opposed to 4.7 percent) were categorized as normal rather than obese.

Taste. While it could of course be true that inconvenience in securing food might preclude the eating behavior of obese persons, it is probably true that other stimulus qualities of food per se also exert strong influences. While it is recognized that taste is a composite evaluation based upon an interaction between such factors as "the affective arousal that follows ingesting of certain foods, or being deprived of them, the existing habits of and attitudes of an organism, and the chemical state of the organism as determined by its constitution and dietary history,"[36] it is nonetheless possible to manipulate the taste of a food through straightforward chemical additions and subtractions as well as through varied forms of processing. Therefore it may not be inappropriate to consider taste to be an external characteristic of food.

Hashim and Van Itallie[37] undertook what has already become a classic study of the effect of taste upon the eating of normal and obese subjects studied at the Nutrition Clinic of Saint Luke's Hospital in New York. They obtained estimates of the pre-experimental eating by their paid subjects, finding the obese group reporting the consumption of an average of 3,500 calories per day as opposed to the 2,200 calories for the nonobese subjects. Upon admission to the ward, the obese subjects were fed, for successive weeks, 2,400 then 1,200 calorie diets while the normal subjects consumed a normal 2,400 calorie diet during the two-week period. During the experimental period, all subjects were offered a bland, nutritionally sound but comparatively untasty liquid diet. While the normal subjects continued to consume a normal amount of the liquid, the obese subjects diminished their intake to an average of 500 calories per day for the three-week duration of the study. The authors quite correctly concluded from their observations that obese persons are more influenced by the taste of the food which they eat than are nonobese individuals.

Nisbett undertook two further studies of the effect of taste manipulation upon the eating of obese persons. Subjects in the first of these studies,[38] believing that they were participating in a study of the effects of hunger upon concentration, were asked to skip the meal prior to the experiment. After filling out some questionnaires, one half of the subjects were given an opportunity to eat roast beef and Swiss cheese sandwiches while one half of the subjects were given no food. Then both groups were asked to sample ice cream from a container introduced to them as "bitter vanilla." One sample of the ice cream was commercially available sweet vanilla while the other was doctored with the addition of 2.5 grams of quinine sulphate per quart. The results, determined by the number of grams of ice cream which each subject consumed, firmly support the hypothesis that overweight subjects will be more influenced by taste than will normal-weight subjects. When they liked the ice cream, as some members of both groups did, obese subjects were likely to eat more of it than the nonobese controls independently of whether they were first fed sandwiches. In discussing his own data, Nisbett raised another intriguing question — he wondered whether the observed eating was a consequence of weight or a cause of weight. He found a partial answer to this question by investigating the amount of ice cream eaten by those normal subjects who had histories of being overweight. With an almost eerie concordance with the hypothesis, he found that "subjects with a history of overweight ate more good ice cream and less bad ice cream than those without such a history."[39]

To generalize this finding further, Nisbett showed that "what's true for ice cream is apparently also true for cake."[40] Working with Drs. Harry Jacobs and Joel Sidel, he investigated the responses of volunteer cake tasters at the U.S. Army Laboratories at Natick, Massachusetts. Volunteers were asked to rate on a nine-point scale cakes which ranged from the finest available to cake which was stored at 100° for 100 days. As in the ice cream study, the results indicated that:

> Underweight subjects ate more disliked cake and less extremely liked cake than normal subjects. Overweight subjects ate roughly the same amount of disliked cake as other subjects but considerably more of the cake which they liked. Again, the response of the overweight subjects was an "on-off" character. Nearly all of the slope occurs across the middle of the range of evaluations.[41]

Finally, Decke also found that what is true for cake and ice cream is also true for milk.[42] According to Schachter, she found that while normal subjects drank more vanilla milk shake with good taste (10.6 ounces) than with quinine taste (6.4 ounces), obese subjects averaged 13.9 ounces of good milk shake as opposed to 2.6 ounces of quinine-treated milk shake.

Above and beyond these studies which show that the taste effect generalizes across foods for the obese person, Goldman, Jaffa, and Schachter [43] in the study mentioned earlier, showed that obese students have a higher probability of putting their money where their taste buds lead them. Working again with undergraduates at Columbia University who had a choice of fulfilling meal contracts and taking their meals from institutional kitchens on campus or canceling their meal contracts in favor of foraging for their meals in off-campus restaurants at a penalty of $15, the researchers showed — as one might have expected by now — that 86.5 percent of the fat freshmen canceled their meal contracts as compared with 67.1 percent of the normal freshmen. Therefore taste is again shown to be a factor which exerts a stronger influence upon obese individuals as opposed to those of normal weight.

Taken together, these studies can be understood to have at least partially substantiated the notion that taste, as a selected characteristic of food and also a factor with a locus in the external environment, may exert a greater influence upon the eating of obese people than their internal physiological state. Following from this, however, it is appropriate to wonder whether other internal reactions such as emotions might not exercise the same cue value in eating as do external events. This assumption is particularly attractive in light of findings of some of the psychological writers such as Simon who suggested that obese persons tend to be depressed.[44] If obese individuals have a disproportionate tendency to be unhappy, then one may wonder whether unhappiness may not be a trigger for eating.

Emotional state. As a means of exploring the effect of emotional state upon eating, Drs. Schachter, Goldman, and Gordon[45] again resorted to deception. Asking subjects not to eat before the experiment, they offered one half of the subjects a roast beef sandwich and a glass of water, offering the other subjects none. Then members of each group were shown a large imposing console of electronic gear, one half being told that they would be exposed to severe shock in a test of the interaction between stimulation and taste, the other being told that they would experience at most a slight tingle. Both groups were then asked to taste and rate crackers for a fifteen-minute period prior to the shock condition. Shock was subsequently not administered, the data supporting the hypothesis derived from observations of the cracker eating under the conditions of food deprivation or nondeprivation, high fear (severe shocks) or low fear (mild shocks). The results indicated that whereas one group of normal-weight subjects (low fear, deprivation) ate almost twice the number of crackers as those in the remaining three groups, the obese subjects ate slightly but not significantly more crackers during the high fear condition, suggesting an interaction between emotional state and eating existed for normal but *not* for obese subjects. Moreover, to make this finding even more interesting, the obese subjects actually reported more fear than the normal-weight group. Analyzing the reactions of their subjects still further, the authors showed that anxiety and nervousness about shock decreased more for normal than obese subjects following eating, therefore leading to a refutation of the commonplace ideas that obese individuals are more likely to eat in response to negative arousal than are normal persons and that eating is more likely to reduce the discomfort of obese persons than of normal persons.

As suggested earlier, complicated designs which involve deception are likely to be subjected to the possibility of spurious results, a possibility which would arise if the deception were less than totally effective. In an otherwise careful study, Schachter, Goldman, and Gordon neglected to ask one critical question of their subjects: How convinced were you that you would be shocked — i.e., how well were you deceived? In a doctoral dissertation at New York University, Edward H. Conrad[46] attempted to correct this flaw. Working with 108 undergraduates divided into obese and normal samples, Dr. Conrad exposed one third of his subjects to either strong social rejection, a neutral social response, or strong social acceptance. Each of these conditions was achieved through giving the subject false social feedback while he worked at the completion of a "market survey." During the experimental period, subjects were incidentally given an opportunity to eat any of several foods. Contrary to the results of the previous study, Conrad's obese subjects were shown to eat more if they were rejected (followed by the accepted, then the neutral condition) while conversely the normal subjects tended to eat less under the rejection condition (followed by the neutral, then the accepted condition). Therefore while partially refuting the conclusions of the first study, this research shows that both normal and obese subjects are influenced by emotional states although in opposing ways when the arousal is negative, and further that the obese are less likely to eat a great deal when they are not in a state of arousal.

One aspect of Conrad's design was careful attention paid to the reported feelings of his subjects. While the results of these analyses were essentially inconsequential, one very apparent finding was presented. Obese subjects in the rejection condition reported a sharp decrease in boredom after eating in contrast to the normal subjects whose boredom was reported to increase after eating. Therefore Conrad's research, as opposed to that of Schachter, Goldman, and Gordon, would seem to indicate some support for a psychogenic theory of obesity as eating occurred in response to a high arousal state and served effectively to counter boredom, a state of under-arousal.

It is not unusual in the development of science for researchers to arrive at opposing conclusions, and the explanations for contrasting results are myriad. Researchers sampling different subjects, using different research designs, implemented by different experiments using different measurement devices at different times in the testing of variously stated hypotheses, might almost be expected to reach different conclusions. When several investigators concur, in the face of the forces which would seem to compel their arriving at different conclusions, the research worker can have greater confidence in the conclusion.

While not manipulating eating per se, the work of Rodin[47] contributes data to the question of the role of environmental factors in eating. She was concerned with whether obese individuals are drawn to environmental cues of food rather than being attracted by any salient environmental stimulus. To find an answer to this question she asked obese and nonobese people to engage in a proofreading task. She asked both groups to work under one of four conditions: no distraction or while listening to one of three audio tapes ranging from neutral discussion about rain or seashells to discussions of the Hiroshima bombing or the subject's own death. She postulated that the obese persons would be more readily distracted and found that not only were the obese subjects more distractable but they were also better proofreaders when distraction was minimal. On the other hand, while the accuracy of the obese subjects fell following the introduction of a more compelling stimulus, the accuracy rate for nonobese persons rose in the face of competing distracting cues. Therefore from these data she concluded that obese and normal subjects differ in at least two ways: their weight and the fact that the obese group is more "stimulus bound" — i.e., more likely to attend to pressing details either of a neutral task or in an emotionally charged background.

In related studies, Drs. Schachter, Rodin, and Herman[48] showed that obese persons were able to recall more detail from slides which they viewed briefly and were also faster in measures of complex (although not simple) reaction time as contrasted with nonobese persons. The simple reaction time measures were taken by asking subjects to lift their finger from a telegraph key upon the appearance of a stimulus light while complex reaction time was measured by asking subjects to lift their left index finger upon the appearance of the right light and vice versa. All of these studies, taken together, would seem to suggest that obese persons who are often termed "hypersensitive" may indeed be just that — they may respond more precisely to the cues for eating or not eating found in the environment, suggesting strongly that while obesity may be psychogenic in origin, it can be controlled through manipulation of environmental events.

Feedback and competing cues. Exploration of the interaction between internal state (e.g., hunger) and external conditions (e.g., feedback and competing cues) can shed light upon the implications of the finding that obese persons are more stimulus bound than nonobese persons. If feedback is a type of information about one's own behavior (e.g., how close one progresses toward a goal), then it would be profitable to investigate the effect which feedback about the amount eaten has upon the rate of eating. Such a line of investigation would supply a dimension missing from the studies of Schachter and Nisbett who carefully manipulated feedback about the amount eaten by their subjects in the service of deception. Goldman[49] utilized what may be a classic design in evaluating the importance of feedback. Feeding his subjects milk shakes which they drank through straws from a gallon container marked in ounces, he controlled feedback simply by allowing or not allowing subjects to see the container. The data revealed that obese subjects drank less when they could see how much they drank than when they could not exactly monitor their intake. Furthermore, Goldman's data showed that normal-weight subjects behaved in exactly the reverse manner, drinking less when they could not discern the exact amount of their intake and more when they did have exact information. Therefore this study showed that when obese subjects have two sources of information — internal cues of hunger and external cues such as feedback — the latter, external force will have a more direct effect upon the rate of their eating than the former, internal cue.

In an unpublished study, Stuart attempted to determine whether the source of feedback was important to obese and normal subjects. He asked 100 students at the University of Michigan, one half of whom were 15 percent or more overweight, to participate in an evaluation of audio tapes presenting arguments favoring the legalization of marijuana and abortion. Subjects were told that because this project was not sponsored research they unfortunately could not be paid in any way other then being offered a chance to help themselves from a bowl of various types of cookies. Designed to evaluate the effect of feedback induced by self or others, immediately or afterward, the subjects, who were seen in groups of three pairs for a 15-minute session, were given one of five sets of instructions at the beginning of the session. They were told to:

1. Do nothing but concentrate on the arguments; there was no further mention of food.

2. Keep track of the number of cookies they ate by marking a 3 x 5 notecard whenever they ate a cookie.

3. Keep track of the number of cookies their partner ate by marking a 3 x 5 notecard when the partner ate a cookie, so that each knew his eating was being socially monitored.

4. Record at the conclusion of the session the number of cookies they had eaten.

5. Record at the conclusion of the session the number of cookies they thought their partner had eaten.

Meanwhile, the experimenter recorded surreptitiously the actual number of cookies eaten by each subject using a concealed button-operated recorder. Bearing in mind that the study manipulated cognitive variables so that the subjects believed that they were earning cookies as payment for participation in research, it is first of interest to determine whether obese subjects were more vulnerable to the "demand charactersitics" of the situation. Controlling for the length of time since the last meal, Stuart found that the overweight students *did not* eat more than the normal-weight students, although they did eat more when time since the last meal was not controlled. More to the point, however, he found the following average consumption of cookies for each of the feedback conditions:

	Overweight	Normal Weight
No feedback	10.3	7.0
Self-recording, immediate	7.2	5.4
Self-recording, delayed	9.8	6.1
Other recording, immediate	3.1	5.9
Other recording, delayed	6.2	6.2

From these data it should be clear that both overweight and normal-weight subjects ate more cookies when no feedback was offered. For normal subjects no significant differences followed from any of the other manipulations, seeming to indicate that these subjects ate what they thought they should independent of the monitoring conditions. For overweight subjects, on the other hand, social (other) monitoring was far more effective in curbing eating than self-recording, and immediate feedback proved superior to delayed feedback in both self- and other monitoring conditions.

Understood in the light of the view that obese persons are generally more stimulus bound than persons of normal weight, the data developed by Goldman and Stuart seem to indicate that when external cues to stop or temper eating are available, overweight subjects will behave in deference to those cues rather than in response to any visceral cues. Conversely, one may speculate that in the absence of such external cues to moderate eating or to attend to stimuli other than food-relevant events, it is possible that obese persons may eat in a problematic fashion. It is suggested that this constellation of events may explain the "night-eating syndrome" which Stunkard found to be characterized by:

> ... morning anorexia, evening hyperphagia, and insomnia. It occurs during periods of life stress and is often alleviated with reduction of the stress. Investigation has thus far failed to establish any consistent personal meaning of either the morning anorexia or the evening hyperphagia, in the sense that they constitute a symbolic representation or resolution of a conflict. Furthermore, persons manifesting this syndrome generally express little self-condemnation that is related to their overeating.[50]

If the view presented here is correct, morning anorexia may be a consequence of the availability of social encounters and experiences which counter the stimulus value of food while evening hyperphagia may result from the absence of external cues which would reduce the rate of eating.

Other research may also be cited in support of this supposition. For example, Taggart[51] reported an eleven-week study of the food intake/weight ratio of one woman, whose weight between weeks was stable over the entire period but with marked and consistent fluctuations within each seven-day period. Although she consumed an average of 2,300 calories

Monday through Friday during which time she lost a slight amount of gross weight, on Saturdays and Sundays she ate an average of 2,580 and 3,050 calories respectively, thereby regaining her temporarily lost weight. Thus she entered the weekend with a 700-calorie energy deficit, without feeling hungry, but gradually recovered the deficit over the weekend. During the weekends she presumably (a) had greater opportunity to eat, and (b) was exposed to fewer competing stimuli. It is suggested, in light of this evidence, that the night-eating syndrome is in effect a diurnal microcosm of the weekly eating patterns of Everyman and is potentially controllable through manipulation of the conditions under which it occurs.

Finally, while it may be stretching the point, it is also possible to use the same explanation for the other problematic eating patterns identified by Stunkard — "binge eating" in which "enormous amounts of food may be consumed in relatively short periods,"[52] and "eating-without-satiation" in which the overeater "experiences difficulty in stopping eating once he has started, without, however, having shown any prior increase, either in the intensity of feelings of hunger or in the desire to eat."[53]

OF MICE AND MEN

In the first section of this chapter it was asserted that although psychologically oriented theories are the most common explanations of overeating, they may not be as fruitful as the behavioral theories which were reviewed in the second part of this chapter. To keep the relationship between the two approaches clear, it may be said that while the behavioral approach does not refute the accuracy of the psychological approach, it does, as will be shown in the next chapter, offer the promise of interventions which have proven to be more effective in shorter times of treatment than is true for intervention following from the psychological view.

In a sense, the contrast between the two explanations of overeating might be viewed as an effort to determine the relative salience of internal as opposed to external forces in generating and maintaining patterns of problematic eating. Paralleling the concern with psychogenic eating in men, various investigators have explored the neurophysiological precursors of inappropriate eating in mice. Beginning with the work of Dr. Neal Miller and his associates (Drs. C.J. Bailey and J.A.F. Stevenson),[54] various researchers have been concerned with the eating behavior of rats, cats, mice, monkeys, and other infrahuman species when these animals have undergone experimental surgery which involves bilateral lesions in the ventromedial nuclei of the hypothalamus, a sector of the brain believed to control a broad array of functions including consumatory responses such as eating. Observations of these animals reveal that they have a tendency to eat large quantities of food during a dynamic phase of hyperphagia with eating and weight gain leveling off during the static phase. What is of interest about these animals is that their behavior very closely parallels the eating behavior of obese humans[55] in a great many ways including a greater preference for taste, a lowered rate of exercise, a disinclination to eat when the response cost is high, and a tendency toward distractability when compared with normal animals.

The importance of these observations lies in the fact that the animals and men appear to behave in many parallel ways. If the process of science by analogy is acceptable as a source of hypotheses about cross-species comparisons, then it may be reasonable to suppose that the human overeater may overeat because of a hypothalamic deviation affecting many aspects of his activities. If this is true, then it may be proven that the treatment of choice for overeating may be found in surgical or psychopharmacological approaches to the modification of specific neurophysiological mechanisms, should safe, response-specific procedures ever be developed for this purpose. For the present, however, it is appropriate to raise a question: If overeating is a consequence of hypothalamic deviation, must it be supposed that these deviations explain all overeating? The Public Health Service has strongly suggested that obesity may not be a monolithic condition:

> Obesity, the result of a positive caloric balance, can be the outcome of a number of disturbances. The variations in causes and subsequent manifestations indicate that not all obesity can be considered the same. For this reason, some investigators have come to use the plural term "obesities" rather than "obesity."[56]

If this is true, then it is wise to think expansively of multiform and polygenetic types of obesity for which various remedies may be practical. This gives rise to a second question: Are there any common denominators to the currently available range of behavioral techniques for the control of overeating? An effort to partially answer this question will be the object of the following chapter.

FOOTNOTES

1. Mendelson, M. Psychological aspects of obesity. *International Journal of Psychiatry*, 1966, *2*, 599-610.
2. Hamburger, W.W. Emotional aspects of obesity. *Medical Clinics of North America*, 1951, *35*, 483-499.
3. Bruch, H. Transformation of oral impulses in eating disorders: Conceptual approach. *Psychiatric Quarterly*, 1961, *35*, 458-481; and Bruch, H. *The importance of overweight*. New York: Norton, 1957.
4. Deri, S. K. A problem in obesity. In A. Burton and R. E. Harris (Eds.), *Clinical studies in personality*. New York: Harper, 1955. P. 574.
5. Bruch, H. Hunger and instinct. *Journal of Nervous and Mental Disease*, 1969, *149*, 100-101.
6. Bruch, H. Conceptual confusion in eating disorders. *Journal of Nervous and Mental Disease*, 1961, *133*, 46-54.
7. Deri, *op. cit.*
8. Bychowski, G. On neurotic obesity. *Psychoanalytic Review*, 1950, *34*, 318.
9. Kaplan, H.I. and Kaplan, H.S. The psychosomatic concept of obesity. *Journal of Nervous and Mental Disease*, 1957, *125*, 181-201.
10. Simon, R.I. Obesity as a depressive equivalent. *Journal of the American Medical Association*, 1963, *183*, 208-210.
11. Conrad, S.W. The problem of weight reduction in the obese woman. *American Practitioner and Digest of Treatment*, 1954, *5*, 38-47.
12. Stunkard, A. Eating patterns and obesity. *Psychiatric Quarterly*, 1959, *33*, 284.
13. Patterson, G.R. and Bechtel, G.G. Formulation of the situational environment in relation to states and traits. In R.B. Cattell (Ed.), *Handbook of modern personality study*. Chicago: Aldine, 1969.
14. Bruch, H. The psychosomatic aspects of obesity. *American Practitioner and Digest of Treatment*, 1954, *5*, 48-49.
15. Glucksman, M.L., Hirsch, J., McCully, R.S., Barron, B.A., and Knittle, J.L. The response of obese patients to weight reduction: A quantitative evaluation of behavior. *Psychosomatic Medicine*, 1968, *30*, 359-373.
16. *Ibid.*, p. 371.
17. Shipman, W.G. and Plesset, M.R. Anxiety and depression in obese dieters. *Archives of General Psychiatry*. 1963, *8*, 26-31.
18. Cauffman, W.J. and Pauley, W.G. Obesity and emotional status. *Pennsylvania Medical Journal*, 1961, *64*, 505-507.
19. *Ibid.*, p. 506.
20. Stuart, R.B. *Short-term behavior therapy: A text*. Itasca, Ill.: Peacock Publishers, in press.
21. Szasz, T. *The myth of mental illness*. New York: Hoeber-Harper, 1967.
22. Fenichel, O. *The psychoanalytic theory of neurosis*. New York: Norton, 1945.
23. Deri, *op. cit.*, p. 579.
24. Stuart, R.B. *Trick or treatment: How and when psychotherapy fails*. Champaign, Ill.: Research Press, 1970.
25. Stunkard, A. Obesity and the denial of hunger. *Psychosomatic Medicine*, 1959, *21*, 281-289.
26. Schachter, A. and Gross, L.P. Manipulated time and eating behavior. *Journal of Personality and Social Psychology*, 1968, *10*, 98-106.
27. *Ibid.*, p. 99.
28. Nisbett, R.E. Taste, deprivation, and weight determinants of eating behavior. *Journal of Personality and Social Psychology*, 1968, *10*, 107-116.
29. Goldman, R., Jaffa, M., and Schachter, S. Yom Kippur, Air France, dormitory food, and the eating behavior of obese and normal persons. *Journal of Personality and Social Psychology*, 1968, *10*, 117-123.
30. *Ibid.*
31. Ross, L.D. Cue- and cognition-controlled eating among obese and normal subjects. Unpublished doctoral dissertation, Columbia University, 1970.
32. Johnson, W.G. The effect of prior-taste and food visibility on the food-directed instrumental performance of obese individuals. Unpublished doctoral dissertation, Catholic University of America, 1970.
33. Nisbett, *op. cit.*

34. Unpublished study by S. Schachter and L. Friedman. Cited in S. Schachter, Some extraordinary facts about obese humans and rats. *American Psychologist,* 1971, *26,* 135.
35. Unpublished study by S. Schachter, L. Friedman, and P. Handler. Cited in Schacther, *ibid.,* p. 135.
36. Young, P.T. Psychologic factors regulating the feeding process. *American Journal of Clinical Nutrition,* 1957, *5,* 160.
37. Hashim, S.A. and Van Itallie, T.B. Studies in normal and obese subjects with a monitored food dispensary device. *Annals of the New York Academy of Science,* 1965, *131,* 654-661.
38. Nisbett, *op. cit.*
39. *Ibid.,* p. 116.
40. Nisbett, R.E. Eating behavior and obesity in men and animals. Unpublished manuscript. Yale University, p. 8.
41. *Ibid.,* p. 9.
42. Unpublished study by Decke. Cited in S. Schachter, *op. cit.,* p. 131.
43. Goldman, Jaffa, and Schachter, *op. cit.*
44. Simon, *op. cit.*
45. Schachter, S., Goldman, R. and Gordon, A. Effects of fear, food deprivation, and obesity on eating. *Journal of Personality and Social Psychology,* 1968, *10,* 91-97.
46. Conrad, E.H. Psychogenic obesity: The effects of social rejection upon hunger, food craving, food consumption, and the drive-reduction value of eating for obese vs. normal individuals. Unpublished doctoral dissertation, New York University, 1968.
47. Rodin, J. Effects of distraction on performance of obese and normal subjects. Unpublished doctoral dissertation, Columbia University, 1970.
48. Unpublished study by J. Rodin, P. Herman, and S. Schachter. Cited in S. Schachter, *op. cit.,* p. 137.
49. Goldman, R.L. The effects of the manipulation of the visibility of food on the eating behavior of obese and normal subjects. Unpublished doctoral dissertation, Columbia University, 1968.
50. Stunkard, Eating patterns and obesity, *op. cit,,* p. 287.
51. Taggart, N. Diet, activity and body-weight: A study of variations in a woman. *British Journal of Nutrition,* 1962, *16,* 223-235.
52. Stunkard, Eating patterns and obesity, *op. cit.,* p. 289.
53. *Ibid.,* p. 290.
54. Miller, N.E., Bailey, C.J., and Stevenson, J.A.F. Decreased "hunger" but increased food intake resulting from hypothalamic lesions. *Science,* 1950, *112,* 256-259.
55. Schachter, *op. cit.*
56. U.S. Public Health Service, *Obesity and Health.* (USPHS Publication No. 1485) Washington, D.C.: U.S. Government Printing Office, 1966. P. 33.

Chapter 3

THE SITUATIONAL MANAGEMENT OF OVEREATING

It is regrettable that Dr. Edgar Gordon was forced to conclude that much of the effort directed toward weight control can be characterized as "faddism and quackery."[1] This may be due in part to the widespread incidence of obesity, the fact that obese persons are victimized by a deviant status and treated as outcasts, and the fact that eating is such a common behavior, influenced by a complex network of customs and unsupported superstition, that almost anyone can claim to be an expert. Some of the "soft science" approach which Dr. Gordon observed was found to permeate the professional literature dealing with the control of obesity as well as being found in the popular press.

Perhaps the most-often-quoted secondary analysis of research relating to the control of obesity was published in 1959 by Dr. Albert Stunkard and Miss Mavis McLaren-Hume.[2] In this paper the authors set forth several appropriate criteria for evaluating the adequacy of research designs in studies pertaining to obesity treatment. Among these criteria were the specification of individual rates of weight change in addition to or in place of group averages, the reporting of data in such a manner as to reflect the experience of patients who either withdrew from treatment or who were otherwise uncooperative, and the specification of treatment time. Using these unimpeachable criteria, the authors reduced the vast number of weight-control studies to a mere eight which employed an acceptable methodology. Of these, seven reported a maximum of 29 percent of their patients lost 20 pounds or more. Based upon these dismal observations the authors could hardly conclude with very much optimism about the prospects facing a patient entering treatment for obesity. It is therefore particularly gratifying that Dr. Stunkard was among those who recently asserted that "behavior modification represents a significant advance in the treatment of obesity."[3] This approach will be briefly summarized, followed by a review of the research results produced by the application of behavior change techniques to the management of obesity and then by a series of recommendations as to how eating can be brought under situational control based, in large measure, upon the results of these studies.

BASIC ELEMENTS OF BEHAVIOR MODIFICATION

The behavioral approach begins with the assumption that all socially relevant behaviors are learned through, and are maintained through, interaction between the individual and relevant persons and situations in his environment. This major assumption has two immediate implications. First, it implies that the environment rather than the man is the agent of control of human behavior, so that efforts to modify behavior should be addressed to changing the environment rather than the man. Second, it implies that the social situation is as much a repository for the conditions associated with acceptable behavior as for unacceptable or problematic behavior. The former implication focuses the technology upon the valid source of behavioral control. The latter implication establishes the ethics of the approach by reversing the more familiar sequence in which the social unit is credited with the control of desirable behavior while the individual is saddled with responsibility for his own undesirable behavior.

The behavioral approach begins and ends with the measurement of the form and rate of observable behaviors. The form of a behavior is what would be seen if it were stopped by a photograph, the rate is the frequency of a response over time, and its observable characteristic establishes the possibility that it can be measured by persons other than the individual himself. The fact that a behavior is observable creates the opportunity for but does not assure that it will be accurately measured. Eating, for example, is an observable behavior of known form and discernible rate. However, it may not always be accurately recorded. The cookie-counting data in the study by Stuart cited in Chapter 2 is one instance of the mismeasurement of eating behavior. Another illustration is provided by Mayer,[4] who showed that obese patients who claimed not to lose weight when following calorie-restricted diets in the open community were observed to lose weight predictably when admitted to an inpatient service where their eating could be monitored. In light of this kind of finding, behavior modifiers such as Azrin and Powell[5] have adopted the caveat of having other persons monitor (the social monitoring) certain kinds of responses at certain times. Were the target behavior not observable — e.g., thoughts or feelings — such monitoring would be impossible and the credibility of behavior change data would be weak.

After identifying the starting form and rate of an observable target behavior, behaviorists next identify the form and rate at which they would like the behavior to occur, in addition to determining the conditions under which this response is expected to occur. For respondent or reflex behaviors — e.g., mouth watering in association with desirable foods or fear of electric shock — the relevant condition is the stimulus which elicits the response, the eliciting stimulus. The aroma of food or the sight of an electric shocker are illustrative eliciting stimuli, and they can be expected to evoke responses of varying magnitudes almost any time they are presented, depending upon factors such as their intensity.

For operant or voluntary behaviors, two sets of conditions are relevant. One set of operant conditions precedes the response. There are four classes of these response "antecedents":

1. Discriminative stimuli are cues which have been associated with some behavioral consequence in the past — e.g., the appearance of a spouse who has consistently praised forebearance — and stimuli delta are cues which have not been associated with such consequences in the past — e.g., the appearance of a stranger. Both sets of cues, therefore, gain their significance through prior learning.

2. Facilitating stimuli are conditions which ease or facilitate the occurrence of the response. Some of these stimuli are the tools necessary for the response — e.g., provision of enough money so that the proper foods can be purchased—while others are the skills which are prerequisites to the response — e.g., a knowledge of acceptable techniques of food preparation.

3. Instructional stimuli are the verbal cues for a response. These cues set forth the rules wherein the behaver learns what consequences to expect from each class of responses— e.g., the instruction that meals are to be served at regular times is a cue that control over the environmental conditions of eating will occur.

4. Potentiating stimuli are the actions taken before a response occurs to strengthen the value of the consequences of that response. For example, a husband can potentiate the value of an evening out for his weight-losing wife if he spends social evenings with her only on the condition that she first follow a prescribed exercise regimen for a period of several days.

Antecedent conditions set the occasion for the occurrence of certain classes of responses. These conditions do not guarantee that the response will in fact occur but they do increase the likelihood of its occurrence.

Consequent conditions are the events which follow and are produced by operant responses. For example, if an overweight man does elect to refuse an offer of a piece of cake, his response might be followed by one of four events:

1. His act might be positively reinforced. That is, someone might do something which he likes, such as praise him or even pay him, thereby strengthening the probability that he will repeat the refusal of cake in the future.

2. His act might be negatively reinforced. That is, his wife might stop nagging him to refuse the cake as soon as he states his refusal. In the future he would be more likely to refuse cake in her presence to the extent that he was relieved by the removal of her nagging.

3. His act might be extinguished. That is, no notice might be taken of his refusal of the cake. In the future he would therefore be less likely to reject cake offers.

4. His act might be punished. That is, he might be denounced as a killjoy or "party pooper" following his refusal. To the extent that these are unpleasant experiences for him, he would be unlikely to pass up cake offers in the company of the same people in the future.

Consequent conditions, then, either accelerate the rate of a response (positive and negative reinforcement) or they decelerate the rate of a response (extinction and punishment).

Some responses produce external environmental change such as the granting or withholding of praise or censure while others produce internal changes such as the building up or satisfaction of an urge to eat. Factors such as the concomitance of external and internal consequences and the regularity (schedule) with which consequences follow responses sometimes make prediction of behavior difficult, but by and large it is correct to say that every socially relevant behavior can be brought under the control of specified antecedent and consequent events. Eating and exercising, as exemplary observable events, are therefore within the purview of control through management of the antecedents and consequences of each.

When a therapist selects a consequence through which to modify the rate of a behavior, he must do so with a view to selecting a strategy which will (a) have the greatest general usefulness, and (b) have the smallest risk of untoward side effects. Changes produced through positive reinforcement are often self-perpetuating because by definition the positively reinforcing consequence has a positive effect upon the rate of the response which produces it. Of course one may tire of positive reinforcements — i.e., one may satiate — but in the natural environment the risks of satiation are small because the person dispensing the positive events can readily either change the regularity with which he delivers a positive reinforcer or he can shift to different kinds of positive reinforcers. Finally, if it is true that the amount of interpersonal attraction which one feels for another is strongly influenced by the strength of the positives received from the other,[6] then use of positive influence techniques can be expected to increase the attraction of the behavior modifier and thereby extend his influence.

Each of the other types of consequences suffers from limitations to which positive reinforcement is immune. With negative reinforcement, the behavior modifier must behave unpleasantly in order to be able to terminate his aversive behavior when a desired response is emitted. But to the extent that he is aversive he will be unpleasant to the other and hence he can expect a decrease in the scope of his influence. Much the same limitation is associated with punishment, for its use also entails the use of aversive manipulations. Punishment is in fact found to be associated with aggression against the punishing agent (operant aggression) or aggression against any innocent bystander (reflexive aggression). Moreover it suffers from the added disadvantages of being extremely difficult to use effectively in the open environment. For punishment to be used with success, fourteen conditions must be fulfilled including the punishment of every problematic behavior, the use of severely aversive consequences, and the delivery of these consequences immediately following a problematic response.[7] Few, if any, of these requirements can be met in the average family, community school, or other nonresearch or noninstitutional environments. Finally, extinction, which requires that only neutral consequences be allowed to follow a behavior, is difficult to engineer. In the normal open community it is often difficult for troublesome behaviors to be ignored either because they are disruptive or because they are reinforced by others. In addition, the use of extinction is likely to reduce the value of the positive reinforcers delivered and therefore is unlikely to be associated with a strong positive attraction between the behaver and the behavior modifier.

Based upon the foregoing arguments, it can be asserted that the use of positive reinforcement strategies is the preferred influence strategy. Beyond the practical reasons for this — it is more generally useful and comparatively risk-free — it can also be asserted that the use of positive influence techniques is more ethically sound than would be the use of any of the others. Positive strategies seek to aid the individual to find ways of increasing his positive outcomes. Two of the other procedures (extinction and punishment) seek to reduce the range of positive reinforcement received by the behaver insofar as they seek to delete from his repertoire responses associated with positively reinforcing consequences. For example, a child who persistently overeats and is "punished" may be required to forego an important pleasure with nothing restored in its place, thereby undergoing a net reduction in the range of his pleasures. In the same vein, negative reinforcement has an adverse effect upon the balance of reinforcements as it adds negative experiences.

To the extent that behavior management is committed to the promotion of human happiness, the use of deceleration strategies should be infrequent. These can sometimes be fruitfully used, as in means of gaining the attention of autistic children participating in self-care or language training,[8] but efforts to decelerate behavior are all too common. It is unfortunate that many professionals, parents, and teachers overlook this ethical principle in managing the behavior of their charges, as demonstrated by the fact that so much professional and lay behavior control is exercised in the service of decreasing the occurrence of problematic behaviors rather than in efforts to increase desirable behaviors. Fortunately, a positive and effective strategy is available in the form of strengthening desirable behaviors which are incompatible with those to be eliminated — as is seen in the effect of reinforcement delivered for appropriate nutritional planning instead of ridiculing poor food choices — and this approach will be shown to be the treatment of choice with obesity.

BEHAVIORAL CONTROL OF OVEREATING

Following pioneering theoretical breakthroughs beginning in the 1920's by such psychological giants as Pavlov, Thorndike, and Skinner, behavior modification approaches began to flourish during the late 1950's. The early behavior modification efforts were largely concerned with the problems of controlling reflexive behavior in accord with the work of Pavlov, these efforts being joined later by efforts to control voluntary behavior aimed at producing a change in the environment. The reflex-oriented strategies were interested in one of two problems. They were either concerned with fostering a negative reaction to events which were positively valued by the individual — e.g., overcoming addictions to alcohol — or they were interested in enabling individuals to overcome maladaptive fears such as fears of heights, closed places, or sex. The operant therapists were interested in a broader spectrum of problems including the replacement of hallucinatory behavior in so-called "schizophrenics" with socially appropriate behavior, the replacement of criminal acts with socially acceptable behaviors such as work and school attendance by delinquents, the enhancement of learning by mental defectives, and the enhancement of marital and family functioning. The literature on behavior modification addressed to the treatment of obesity can similarly be divided into these two categories — respondent and operant approaches.

Respondent treatments. Respondent treatments involve the pairing of one event which has positive value with one which has negative value. The goal of this pairing of two stimuli of unlike value is either to create a positive reaction to a previously negative stimulus — like pairing relaxation with thoughts about fear-arousing social encounters — or to create a negative reaction to previously positive stimuli, like pairing electric shock with the visualization or taste of problematic foods.

Respondent conditioners have paired four types of aversive stimuli with desired foodstuffs in an effort to weaken individuals' attraction to these foods. The first stimulus is electric shock. One of the first, if not the first effort to manipulate food choice in humans with shock was undertaken by F.A. Moss in 1924.[9] A blindfolded child was fed orange juice on some trials and vinegar on others. The child willingly accepted the orange juice but rejected the vinegar. When a clicking noise which had been paired with the vinegar on the early trials was sounded in association with the orange juice on later trials, the orange juice too was rejected. This is a demonstration of aversive conditioning for it entailed training the child in a negative reaction to a stimulus which had a positive value prior to training.

This same procedure has been used in various forms with patients presenting different kinds of problems. Dr. Joseph Wolpe[10] delivered electric shocks to an obese woman when she indicated that she thought about troublesome foods. Following several sessions of this training, the woman reported feeling fearful and/or revolted by thoughts of these foods in the natural environment. Wolpe's patient began to lose weight using this procedure but treatment was terminated when she died due to unrelated causes. Meyer and Crisp[11] later used a similar procedure with two female inpatients. A 26-year-old woman who was obese and addicted to amphetamines, ostensibly to reduce her weight, and a 51-year-old hypochondriacal mother of five were offered treatment which consisted of delivering electric shocks for actually approaching foods which each regarded as especially tempting. The first woman received five shocks during the first session and did not approach the tempting food again over thirty sessions. Her weight fell appreciably during treatment and remained low at a follow-up evaluation almost two years later. The second woman refused to accept a second shock, thereby terminating treatment. Her weight was increased at the time of follow-up.

Each of the foregoing studies was an uncontrolled case report. Studies designed in this manner are useful for generating hypotheses about possible effective interventions, but validation of these hypotheses depends upon the replication of carefully designed research. Stollak[12] improved upon the methodology of these when he attempted to validate the effectiveness of shock to curb problematic eating approach behaviors through a controlled investigation. Working with 138 subjects, not all of whom were randomly assigned to different experimental conditions, Stollak offered six types of treatment: contact control, no-contact control, no-contact diary, contact diary, contact diary-nonspecific shock, and contact diary/shock with food association. The control conditions involved obtaining no more than before-after weight measurements. The diary conditions asked subjects to record their food intake, and the shock conditions involved delivering electric shock either in association with or not in association with food-relevant conversation during treatment sessions. Results unfortunately failed to include the scores of 39 subjects who discontinued treatment but reflected a clear superiority of the contact-diary condition in which subjects recorded their eating behavior and discussed their diaries for 15 minutes per week for several weeks. Of the two shock conditions, the delivery of shock not associated with food conversation resulted in an average one pound gain while the shock-contingent condition resulted in an average 2.9 pound loss.

The second type of aversive stimulus used to weaken the appeal of foods is bad odor. Kennedy and Foreyt[13] worked with a 29-year-old 322-pound woman who had failed in numerous prior attempts to lose weight. They fitted her with a gas mask during treatment sessions. One tube into the mask carried the aroma of her favorite foods. This tube could be closed off by a stopcock which opened another tube carrying the putrid odor of butyric acid. During 22 weeks of treatment she lost 30 pounds, her lowest weight of 284 pounds being recorded at the thirteenth week, after which her weight rose slightly.

The third technique, "covert sensitization," was developed by Dr. Joseph Cautela.[14] In this procedure, subjects are asked to imagine that they are about to eat a problematic food and then to switch immediately to thoughts about unpleasant events, e.g., vomiting or infidelity by a spouse. For a small number of clinical patients, moderate success has been claimed for this procedure.[15]

The fourth type of aversive condition used was breath holding as employed by Tyler and Straughan.[16] These researchers compared three techniques — breath holding being the aversive procedure. Of the 57 subjects in this experiment, one third were assigned to a condition in which they were asked to begin holding their breath as soon as they had thoughts about problematic foods and their appeal. In theory, some of the unpleasantness associated with the breath holding was expected to be attributed (conditioned) to the thoughts about food. After nine weeks of treatment, the subjects in this condition were found to have lost an average of just .43 pounds.

As can be seen from the above summaries, the results associated with the use of deconditioning procedures designed to break down the pairing between positive reactions and problematic foods have been poor. Whether the targets are experimental subjects or clinical patients, the reaction to intervention is generally negative and the results of treatment are disappointing. This may in part be due to the fact that punishment leads to highly discriminative control over behavior, that is, one learns to suppress the response primarily in the presence of the punishing agent, the problematic response recurring in his absence. As a second explanation, it is also possible that the act of eating is so strongly positively reinforcing that the minor inconvenience or discomfort associated with aversive intervention may be trivial when compared with the great pleasure associated with eating. A third explanation for the failure of aversive procedures may be the assumption that eating is or could be brought under essentially personal control. As was stated in Chapters 1 and 2, there is good reason to reject efforts to explain the origin or maintenance of any behavior by reference to internal state. These results contribute to such a rejection.

Efforts to condition positive reactions to desirable foods have yielded a mixed outcome. The last study mentioned, the work of Tyler and Straughan,[17] compared a positive conditioning program with the aversive technique and a "relaxation" control group. In the positive conditioning paradigm, Homme's coverant control technique[18] was used. Homme regards coverants as "covert operants" or cognitive behaviors. He believes that they can be controlled in much the same manner as can any other behavior and set about to demonstrate this by arranging for his subjects to think specific thoughts immediately prior to engaging in their own choice of pleasurable behaviors occurring frequently throughout the day. For example, his subjects might be directed to think about eating desirable foods just prior to taking a drink of water or sitting down each day. In this manner the positive value of drinking and sitting is expected to condition thoughts of appropriate food choices. Regrettably the subjects undergoing this treatment in the Tyler and Straughan study lost only .75 pounds during the nine weeks of treatment.

While the Tyler and Straughan study helps to refute the feasibility of conditioning even positive changes, a recent study by Horan[19] who worked with 96 undergraduate women at Michigan State University reached a more affirmative conclusion. Horan "impartially" (randomly?) assigned his subjects to one of four experimental conditions, three of which were controls for the main condition in which the Homme procedure was followed. Over eight weeks, subjects in the main experimental condition lost an average of 5.66 pounds in contrast to 3.13 and 2.72 pounds lost by the two closest control groups.

The Horan study is unusual in two respects. First it reports the data for every subject, and from these data it is evident that 12 of 19 subjects in the focal treatment lost more weight (one subject losing 19.25 pounds) than the average subject in the more effective control, while four subjects gained weight (one subject gaining 8.25 pounds). These data reflect the fact that overweight people are likely to be highly individualistic in their response to any particular procedure. The data also suggest that much of the group difference is attributable to several subjects who gained or lost weight dramatically and that more factors than just the coverant control procedure—e.g., experimenter influence in the form of the expectancy of more positive outcome for one as opposed to the other groups—may have contributed to the superiority of the focal treatment. The second factor which distinguishes this study is that Horan presented data showing the extent to which subjects in the two most closely related conditions reported that they followed the experimental prescription. It will be seen

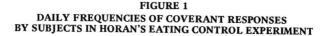

FIGURE 1
DAILY FREQUENCIES OF COVERANT RESPONSES
BY SUBJECTS IN HORAN'S EATING CONTROL EXPERIMENT

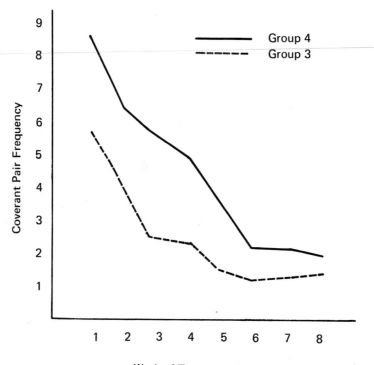

Reproduced with permission from J. J. Horan, The effect of coverant conditioning on weight reduction. Paper presented at the annual meeting of the American Educational Research Association, 1971.

in Figure 1 that over time there was a steady decrease in the extent to which the procedures were used. Other studies[20] have shown that weight loss is most likely to occur at the start of treatment. Viewed in the perspective of Horan's data, this early weight loss and later plateau may be attributable to a greater likelihood that prescriptions will be followed early as opposed to later in the treatment.

In summary, it can be said that efforts to decondition the association between positive reactions and problematic foods have been less successful than efforts to condition positive reactions to non-problematic foods.[21] However the results of research using either approach appear to be inconsequential unless some external supports for behavior change are introduced—e.g., experimenter attention. Therefore while conditioned or reflexive reactions to food may be relevant to intervention at this time, it cannot be said that they are sufficient conditions for the change of eating patterns over time.

Operant treatments. Whereas respondent treatments are concerned with training new reactions (reflexes) to eliciting stimuli, operant treatments are concerned with strengthening or weakening existing responses in association with particular antecedent and consequent stimuli. Perhaps because operant conditioners must find the desired response in the repertoire of their patients or subjects, they tend to make more positive assumptions about the relative strengths of their proteges than do respondent conditioners or psychotherapists. This, in turn, may explain the fact that operant conditioning programs are more likely to attend to an increase in the strength of appropriate eating rather than concentrating upon weakening inappropriate eating.

The first in a series of papers on operant methods as applied to overeating was published by Ferster, Nurnberger, and Levitt.[22] Weakened by an absence of data, this paper has served as a cornerstone for the work of many researchers who have applied operant methods successfully with normal and so-called "schizophrenic" overeaters. Ferster and his colleagues directed some effort toward making overeaters aware of the ultimate aversive consequences of overeating—consequences such as illness, loss of loved ones, and the like. Other techniques suggested by these researchers included keeping careful records of food intake, scheduling eating to occur at given intervals, gaining stimulus control of all eating, and strengthening prepotent activities which would be incompatible with eating such as housework or activities occurring outdoors.

The next in this series of papers was the work of Stuart.[23] He applied the paradigm generated by Ferster and his colleagues, with some modifications, to the treatment of eight women whose weight loss over 12 months ranged from 29 to 47 pounds. The treatment used by Stuart was not short in duration, ranging from 19 to 41 sessions, each of which lasted approximately half an hour. Stuart's six-step curriculum involved procedures ranging from the use of Cautela's covert sensitization to the techniques of manipulating the antecedents and consequences of eating as well as changing the act of eating itself. Each of these steps will be fully described in the next section.

Dr. Mary B. Harris[24] undertook the first controlled test of these methods. (The results were compiled in 1967 but not published until 1969.) Working with 24 men and women who were at least 15 pounds overweight and who answered an advertisement in the Stanford University newspaper, she assigned her subjects to either of two experimental sections or to a control group. The experimental sections both offered treatment which had, essentially, three components: (1) training in the concepts of reinforcement in which, for example, "suggestions were made as to methods useful for making reward for refraining from eating more immediate . . . ";[25] (2) analysis of the stimuli controlling eating behavior, leading to suggestions as to how to reduce the likelihood of problematic eating, for example, by not walking past candy machines; and (3) slowing the rate of eating by, for example, training subjects to swallow the last bite before putting more food into their mouths. After a period of 10 weeks in which treatment was conducted on a group basis, one half of the experimental subjects were placed in an aversive conditioning program using Cautela's covert sensitization. The results of the study were impressive, with the change in weight occurring in the experimental conditions significantly greater than that observed for the control subjects. Furthermore, the difference between the two halves of the experimental group—those which did and did not receive covert sensitization—was nonsignificant, implying that this procedure added little to the outcome.

The next experimental validation of this approach was undertaken as a doctoral dissertation by Dr. Janet P. Wollersheim at the University of Illinois.[26] Dr. Wollersheim's design is the most ambitious to date, involving 79 overweight students observed for 18 weeks of baseline, 12 weeks of treatment (including 10 treatment sessions) and 8 weeks of follow-up. She assigned her subjects to one of four experimental conditions: a group in which social pressure was used to try to induce weight loss (analogous to the TOPS program[27]), a nonspecific treatment group seeking to develop insight into problematic eating, a focal treatment group using many of the operant procedures described above, and an untreated, waiting-list control group. Among these conditions, all three groups outperformed the control group at a significant level, but the focal (operant) treatment significantly outperformed the social pressure and insight group as well. When the responses of individual subjects were studied, it was found that 50, 33, and 21 percent of the subjects respectively in the focal, social pressure, and insight groups lost a significant amount of weight, the average weight loss for the focal group being 9.11 pounds. One disquieting note is found in the fact that the only group failing to show a slight weight gain at follow-up was the insight group, despite the fact that only the focal treatment group reported a systematic decrease in the frequency of problematic eating responses during treatment.

The third controlled study involved a comparison of these operant techniques with a psychotherapeutic group in a clinical setting. Of the foregoing studies, only Stuart worked with a "clinical" as opposed to "experimental" population. Also, in each of the foregoing studies, therapist or experimenter expectancy[28] of outcome might have been expected to have a biasing effect upon outcome, although Wollersheim had each of the therapists involved in each form of intervention. In the study conducted by Drs. Penick, Filion, Fox, and Stunkard[29] at the Department of Psychiatry of the University of Pennsylvania, all patients were seen in a day hospital program for the treatment of obesity. Of the 32 patients, all were at least 20 percent overweight and were either private patients or physical medicine rehabilitation patients. Furthermore, the leader of the group psychotherapy condition was an internist undergoing a psychiatric residency, with long experience in the treatment of obesity and great skill in group psychotherapy, while the leader of the behavior modification condition was an experienced experimental psychologist, thereby equalizing the experimenter expectancy effect. The behavioral program was thorough and innovative, moving beyond the already familiar techniques of the operant control of overeating (the ingenious recommendations of this group will be identified where relevant in the following section), while the psychotherapy group utilized supportive techniques in addition to dieting and nutritional instruction. The results at the time of follow-up, from three to six months after the termination of the three-month treatment, are summarized in Table 1. It can be seen that over twice as many behavior modification as psychotherapy patients lost 40 and 30 pounds, while almost twice as many lost more than 20 pounds. When it is borne in mind that the average medical literature predicts that only 5 percent of the treated patients will lose more than 40 pounds and 25 percent more than 20 pounds, the results found for the behavior therapy group are most remarkable. Finally, it should be pointed out that, as with the subjects treated by Horan, there was considerable variability in the response of patients to behavioral treatment in this study. This supports the notion that the response of individuals will be idiosyncratic and suggests the need to build into all behavior modification approaches a means of adapting the techniques to individual differences.

These five papers constitute a growing body of literature which

TABLE 1

FOLLOW-UP AT 3-6 MONTHS
PERCENT OF GROUPS LOSING SPECIFIED AMOUNTS OF WEIGHT

	Behavior Modification Groups N=15	Control Therapy Groups N=17
More than 40 lbs.	27	12
More than 30 lbs.	40	18
More than 20 lbs.	53	29

Reproduced with permission from S. D. Penick, R. Filion, S. Fox, and A. J. Stunkard, Behavior modification in the treatment of obesity. Paper presented at the annual meeting of the American Psychosomatic Society, Washington, D.C., March 1970.

points strongly toward the effectiveness of operant principles with "normal" overweight persons in the community, some of whom designate themselves as patients without prompting, others of whom designate themselves only as experimental subjects. The generality of the literature can be extended when studies of the use of operant conditioning techniques in work with obese patients in institutional settings is included. The first of these was contained in the work of Ayllon as one of a series of studies conducted at Saskatchewan Hospital.[30] Ayllon manipulated the overeating and food stealing of his patient merely by removing her from the dining room immediately following any inappropriate eating or food-related behavior. Within two days her eating was brought within desirable limits, and over 14 months her weight decreased from 250 to 180 pounds. Harmatz and Lapuc[31] similarly used money to reinforce weight loss by 21 male psychiatric patients at the Northampton Veterans Administration Hospital, demonstrating that the monetarily reinforced patients continued to lose weight four weeks after the termination of the six-week treatment while the diet-only and control-group patients began to regain weight. Equally dramatic results were obtained by Barnard,[32] whose patient progressed from weighing 407 pounds to a weight of 337 pounds over the course of 17 weeks of treatment. This consisted of giving her tokens redeemable like money for achieving weekly weight reduction objectives. In a related effort, Mann[33] at the University of Kansas "contracted"[34] with his nonpsychotic subjects for weight loss on a weekly basis, returning to them personal possessions previously deposited with the experimenter.

In assessing the general results of these treatments, it is wise to bear in mind that many of the studies report only short-term follow-up data (the longest being 12 months as reported by Stuart[35]), that many of the subjects are perhaps a nonstandard clinical sample (with the exception of the work of Penick and his associates[36] and Stuart[37]), and that the number of replications of the techniques using acceptable scientific rigor is as yet small. The significance of the improvement in probable outcome associated with behavioral as opposed to nonbehavioral techniques, however, will certainly stimulate the research which is still needed. This is particularly true in light of two findings related to overall weight loss. First it has been shown that the psychological distress predicted as an accompaniment for weight loss not buffered by psychological treatment has not occurred. Harris, for example, found:

> General level of tension or depression as well as tension specifically related to eating showed only nonsignificant decreases from beginning to end of the experiment and no relationship to the amount of weight loss.[38]

And Wollersheim found that anxiety reduction was in fact related to weight loss in a program which revealed the emergence of no "symptom" substituting for weight.[39] Thus while the depression observed by Stunkard[40] to be associated with weight loss undoubtedly occurred in association with more traditional treatments, it is not found to be associated with behavioral treatment. The failure of this reaction to occur may be a result of the fact that this treatment does not expect and therefore would not inadvertently cue such reactions and/or a consequence of the fact that the client is not asked to modify his behavior while the pathogenic environment continues to work against him. Second, it can be shown that the dropout rate for this treatment compares favorably to earlier treatments. None of the patients of Penick and his associates dropped out,[41] only 4 percent of those of Wollersheim discontinued,[42] and 12.5 percent of Harris' subjects failed to complete treatment.[43] Therefore the effectiveness of weight reduction, the absence of apparent untoward psychological side effects and the great probability of maintaining the overeater in treatment, all commend the energetic adoption of these techniques.

ESTABLISHING BEHAVIORAL CONTROL OF OVEREATING

Based upon the principles of behavior modification, therapists have demonstrated that overeating can be successfully controlled in work with normal and "psychotic" adults in home and institutional settings. The principles used by behavior therapists in their work are available to and in fact are universally used by virtually all people at all times. For example, the woman wishing to write a letter to a friend may put her baby to bed, lower the volume of the television set being watched by her older children, and place pen and paper on a well-lighted spot on a cleared table. In so doing she would eliminate one force incompatible with letter writing (a demanding baby), suppress another (the volume of the television set), and strengthen events compatible with letter writing (the availability of the needed implements). She would concentrate upon making her handwriting legible and on expressing her ideas well and she would write first to those who have answered her letters, saving for much later those who neglected to respond to several letters. She has, then, undertaken the management of her own behavior through controlling the situation in which it occurs. These are the same techniques used by behavior therapists as summarized in Figure 2. They merely call for making certain that the antecedent and consequent events which would impede the occurrence of the desired behavior are suppressed while at the same time strengthening the events likely to be associated with its successful performance. Efforts to manage behavior in this manner call for attention to all three elements of behavior—antecedents, the responses themselves, and consequences.

FIGURE 2
PARADIGM FOR REDUCING THE STRENGTH
OF UNDESIRABLE RESPONSES AND INCREASING
THE STRENGTH OF DESIRABLE RESPONSES

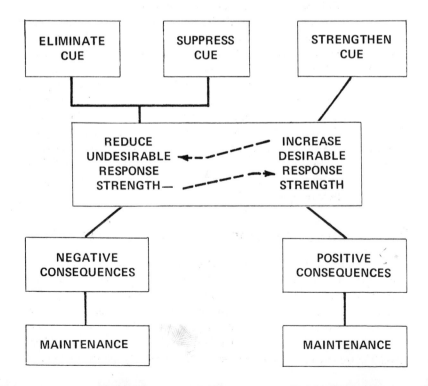

Antecedents. Since the antecedents of a response set the occasion for its occurrence, making it more likely to occur, it stands to reason that one would wish to entirely do away with as many of the cues for problematic behaviors as possible, suppress those which cannot be entirely eliminated, and meanwhile strengthen others which have positive functional value with respect to the achievement of desirable behavioral objectives. In approaching the task of management of the antecedents of problematic and desirable eating responses, it is *first necessary to take a baseline* of the relative frequency of each. To do this, the form in Figure 3 is useful. On this form is recorded much of the information needed for the functional analysis of eating behavior—an analysis of the conditions under which it is likely to occur. For example, the time of eating can provide important cues to the high-risk times of day so that responses which would compete with eating can be planned for those times. Similar use can be made of the data describing the social, physical, and emotional concomitants of problematic eating, for they too serve as a means of identifying the risk conditions with which undesirable eating may be associated. Once the target conditions have been identified, it is possible to plan for the removal of situational forces exercising negative control while strengthening those which should have positive control. This can be achieved through a series of steps leading to the elimination, suppression, or strengthening of selected antecedents.

ELIMINATION STEP ONE

The objective of this step is to facilitate planned control of the antecedents associated with problematic eating. Research dealing with the situational control of hunger and with respondent conditioning procedures provide the rationale for this step. The former group of studies, it will be recalled, demonstrated that obese persons are more vulnerable to external stimulation of hunger and eating responses than nonobese persons. The latter group of studies demonstrated that external cues can acquire relevance to a particular behavior through the process of respondent conditioning in which neutral external events can acquire response-eliciting properties. For example, an obese person who eats in many different environments or who performs many different tasks while eating may come to experience hunger in any environment in which he has previously eaten or may eat in association with any actions with which eating has been associated in the past. When people eat in the living room, office, or bedroom, they are more likely to experience hunger in those rooms than would be true if all of their eating were confined to the kitchen. When they eat while watching television or talking on the phone or playing

FIGURE 3
BASELINE EATING MONITORING FORM

Food eaten		Time	Social		Where eaten	Mood when eaten
Quantity	Type of food	Circle time if food was part of meal	Alone?	With whom?	Home Work Restaurant Recreation	A-Anxious B-Bored C-Tired D-Depressed E-Angry

cards, they may "automatically" become hungry upon undertaking any of these actions. Therefore it is essential to:

ARRANGE TO EAT IN ONLY ONE ROOM

ARRANGE TO EAT AT ONLY ONE PLACE IN THAT ROOM

DO NOT ENGAGE IN ANY OTHER ACTIVITY WHILE EATING

By narrowing the span of situational cues which are associated with eating, the individual has a greatly enhanced possibility of gaining appropriate stimulus control of his behavior. As a measure of the importance of the stimulus control of eating, Dr. Penick and his associates[44] included in their landmark research a requirement that subjects eat on the same distinctively colored placemat whenever they ate, narrowing the scope of cues of eating to the barest minimum. Whether or not this degree of precision is achieved, it is essential for efforts to be made to decondition or dissociate as many irrelevant cues from eating responses as possible in a first step toward gaining appropriate stimulus control.

ELIMINATION STEP TWO

The second step is another in the chain of maneuvers to gain stimulus control. This step calls for putting temptation out of reach. For many persons, eating certain problematic foods has addictive properties. Half gallons of ice cream disappear quickly, bowls of potato chips—as the ads inform us — defy eaters to munch on only one chip, and many foods are marketed in formats which facilitate addictive eating. The best means of dealing with the temptation of such foods is to not purchase them. Therefore it is essential to:

AVOID THE PURCHASE OF PROBLEMATIC FOODS

Food advertisers, packagers, and merchandisers have developed great expertise in creating the desire for foods of little or no nutritional value and which are high in starch and sugar. As a measure of their expertise, the snack food market has grown consistently and has consumed an increasing percentage of the food dollar. When the overeater enters a food store he is entering a contest with a large and powerful industry whose success depends upon his improprieties. His main line of defense therefore is to take whatever steps possible to ensure prudent food selections. One way to do this is *to shop only from a list and to bring into the store only enough money to cover the cost of the necessary purchases.* In this way he can protect himself from seduction by specials on cakes, cookies, soft drinks, and other sweets which would result not only in his buying more, but also in his eating more.

Beyond buying from a list and entering the store with limited money, the overeater can also arrange to do his shopping only after a full meal. Stuart, in an unpublished study, asked twenty obese women who had volunteered for participation in a weight reduction program to do all of their food shopping between the hours of 3:30 and 5:00 p.m., collecting all date-stamped cash register tapes. He asked another group of twenty to do their shopping only between the hours of 6:30 and 8:00 p.m. under the assumption that they would complete their dinner by 6:30. The principal finding in this study was that women who shopped after a full meal purchased a full 19.7 percent less than those who purchased their food prior to eating. To validate this finding the buying time of the two groups was reversed, the before- and after-dinner shoppers exchanging buying times, with a 15.7 percent saving favoring the late shoppers again. This result is the converse of a finding by Nisbett and Kanouse[45] who asked normal and overweight shoppers how long ago they had last eaten and correlated the amount spent on food with the duration of food deprivation. They found that the more deprived shoppers of normal weight bought 43 percent more than did the less deprived nonobese shoppers, but precisely the opposite trend was found for obese women who bought less food if they had been deprived of food longer.

The contrast between the Stuart findings and those of Nisbett and Kanouse vividly points to the kind of conflict which constantly appears in research dealing with obesity. Another manifestation of it is in the conflict between estimates of the effect of eating several small as contrasted with three larger meals. While Gordon repudiated his earlier contention that eating several small meals daily would necessarily result in greater weight loss than eating only three meals,[46] others[47] have shown that with caloric intake held constant, subjects eating seven meals daily lost weight while those eating three maintained their weight. In view of conflicts such as these, it is essential for each would-be weight-loser to attempt to manipulate his behavior toward change in a particular direction. He should then evaluate the effectiveness of the manipulation, and when his observations contrast with the expectations derived from the literature, his experience rather than the literature should be allowed to serve as the guide.

ELIMINATION STEP THREE

The third step toward elimination of the cues of problematic eating is to avoid whenever possible coming into contact with problematic foods which must for some reason be kept in the house. To accomplish this:

DO NOT SERVE HIGH-CALORIE CONDIMENTS AT MEALS

ALLOW CHILDREN AND SPOUSES TO TAKE THEIR OWN SWEETS

CLEAR PLATES DIRECTLY INTO THE GARBAGE

When condiments are served at meals in which they are not an integral part, they are very likely to be eaten indiscriminately not because the overeater is "hungry" but because they are available. To avoid this, high-calorie condiments should not be put on the table. In addition, when children ask for sweets they put their parents into direct contact with foods which might better be avoided. If it is not possible to substitute raisins, nuts, or dates for cookies and candy, it is preferable for children to be asked to take their own sweets in order to avoid the familiar distribution pattern of one for the child, three for the adult. Finally, for more humanitarian reasons—e.g., to protect children in less advantaged circumstances from starvation—adults are likely to eat the table scraps left by their children. Scraping these scraps directly into the garbage will have the same effect as allowing children to take their own sweets—it will eliminate one additional temptation to overeat.

ELIMINATION STEP FOUR

In the foregoing chapter it was shown that obese humans have in common with animals suffering from ventromedial hypothalamic lesions a tendency to not emit complex or difficult responses to obtain food. Therefore the more obstacles that can be placed in the path of free access to food, the less likely it is that the obese person will indulge in problematic eating. Therefore:

MAKE PROBLEMATIC EATING AS DIFFICULT AS POSSIBLE

To do this, those high-calorie foods which are purchased for other family members should only be purchased in a form requiring elaborate preparation—e.g., heating in the oven before serving. When these foods are eaten, they should be prepared only one unit at a time. For example, if the obese person eats bread it should be toasted. If it is toasted, only one slice at a time should be prepared, with the remainder of the loaf being returned to its storage place before eating; and the person should be sitting at the table when that slice of toast is eaten. Therefore in order to eat a second slice he would have to get up from the table, take the bread from its storage place, prepare a slice of toast, return the bread to its storage area, return to the table, sit, and eat the toast. This long chain of responses achieves three purposes: (1) it increases the response cost of eating; (2) it interrupts a process in which "automatic" eating can occur—eating of which the individual may not be fully aware; and (3) it creates a number of choice points at which the individual may choose not to eat.

* * * * *

The first three elimination steps will, if followed, simply reduce the number of opportunities for problematic eating. The fourth step is transitional in nature. If the response cost is sufficiently high, it will eliminate any temptation to eat. However, even if the response cost is not greater than the expected satisfaction derived from eating, this step will nonetheless aid in the suppression of eating if only because of the time delay necessitated by the long chained-response pattern. When cues are suppressed in this manner, they remain present but they do not have the behavioral control strength which would have been present had they not been altered.

SUPPRESSION STEP ONE

Most of the familiar psychological and cultural theories of over-eating, as well as the situational view expressed here, identify social interactional factors as having crucial etiological and maintenance significance for problematic eating patterns. That is, most authors agree that the time and place at which eating occurs, the nature of the food eaten, its manner of preparation, the way in which it is eaten, and the amount eaten, among other things, are patterns learned through a complex process of socialization and are maintained through intricate modes of social interaction. Therefore any effort to suppress eating behavior which is problematic must *first* attend to the social interactional exchanges which both produced and maintain it. Failure to attend to social factors, as in interventions that deal solely with pharmacological and diet regimens self-administered by the overeater, may in effect ask the overeater to modify his behavior while the pathogenic shaping influences continue to operate unchecked. As an example, many a would-be weight-loser embarks upon a program of stoic self-denial only to be greeted by her husband's surprise gift of a five-pound box of chocolates. To reject the offering is to court social disaster; to accept the offering is to surely invite physical disaster. The only viable alternative, therefore, is prophylactic—to prevent the social mismanagement of food:

REPROGRAM THE SOCIAL ENVIRONMENT TO RENDER THE USE OF FOOD AS CONSTRUCTIVE AS POSSIBLE

The concept of "reprogramming the social environment" was first introduced by Dr. G. R. Patterson and his colleagues.[48] They noticed that unless parent-child interactions were modified, changes in the child's behavior produced by conventional therapeutic modes were not successful. They therefore focused their attention upon social interaction in place of the more customary emphasis upon the child's inner dynamics and significantly enhanced treatment outcome and thereby changed the general thrust of services to youth.[49]

In reprogramming the social environment with respect to eating, it is necessary to make two essential changes in a social interactional pattern which is defined as problematic by the obesity of either or both members. The first change is to *provide for positive cueing of desirable behaviors.* By its presence this will serve to suppress some of the antecedents associated with problematic eating, for one cannot both offer food and cue its refusal. The second change is to *provide positive reinforcement for acceptable eating* in the place of the more familiar and more troublesome attacks upon the overeater for errors in his management of food. Strong condemnation for inopportune eating seems to have the effect of increasing tension level and of creating a sense of social injustice, both of which are often requited by eating in the natural course of human behavior. It is only when the cueing of and disproportionate attention to inappropriate eating are replaced by constructive interactions that one can expect appropriate eating patterns to predominate.

As a means of surveillance over the nature of social interaction, it is suggested that both the overeater and at least one salient member of his social environment — spouse, adolescent child, roommate, co-worker, etc. —keep track of the verbal exchanges pertaining to food. This can be readily accomplished by having the overeater record the type of social feedback which he has received as positive or negative, indicating as well whether he did or did not comply with the implied suggestion that he continue or

FIGURE 4
INTERACTION ASSESSMENT FORM

	morning	afternoon	evening
Monday	+ ⊖ +	+ ⊕ +	− ⊖ +
Tuesday			
Wednesday			
Thursday			
Friday			
Saturday			
Sunday			
Total			

discontinue a particular act. The social monitor would be well-advised to keep a similar record of his own behavior, recording the number of occasions upon which he gave positive or negative feedback and whether the message resulted in compliance. The records can be kept on any convenient form, a 3 x 5 index card being ideal for the purpose if ruled as in Figure 4. A plus (+) on the card indicates positive feedback, a minus (−) indicates negative feedback. A circle around the plus or minus indicates noncompliance. A total of the number of the positive and negative, compliance and noncompliance occurrences each day is a clue to the general valence of the interaction. The most acceptable interactions show a significant outbalance of positive over negative interchanges. Feedback such as this can be most helpful in efforts to change a pathogenic social interchange to a highly constructive exchange through providing feedback about patterns of which neither party might be aware.

SUPPRESSION STEP TWO

It has often been observed that when people are alone their social behavior is more crude than when they are in social situations. This is as true for eating as it is for other social exchanges. For example, one question of the Minnesota Multiphasic Personality Inventory asks whether the respondent uses the same table manners at home as in public. An affirmative answer to this question is interpreted as an index of the dishonesty of the respondent. This tendency to be on "good behavior" when in the eye of the public can have an extremely desirable effect upon patterns of overeating. Therefore, whenever possible the overeater should:

HAVE OTHERS MONITOR EATING PATTERNS

The presence of company has the effect of introducing the highest possible level of social control upon eating. Mayer[50] has observed that highly obese patients who claimed to maintain their weight on what would be an anorexogenic diet for a canary lost weight rapidly upon admission to a nutrition ward where their eating could be held to the self-reported level. This same monitoring, when applied to eating in the natural environment, can have the effect of holding down problematic eating, particularly when the social monitor knows that the overeater has committed himself to a program of dietary restriction.

SUPPRESSION STEP THREE

The elimination steps were all designed to enable the overeater to avoid the seduction inherent in the availability of large amounts of problematic food. There are times, however, when one cannot avoid having contact with such food and the temptation must be escaped rather than avoided, escape implying that the exposure to problematic foods has already taken place. At these times it is necessary to:

MINIMIZE CONTACT WITH EXCESSIVE FOOD

There are two ways in which this rule can be followed. First it is helpful for food to be *served on plates in measured small quantities* rather than being served in serving pieces on an *ad lib* basis. Second, it is important for the dieter to *leave the table soon after he finishes his meal,* even if this means getting up after an entree only to return later for dessert. A great many calories are consumed in "picking" at food while others who eat more slowly are finishing their meals. This picking is both unnecessary and problematic and therefore should be inhibited as much as possible.

SUPPRESSION STEP FOUR

In the preceding chapter it was shown that considerable evidence has been adduced in support of the fact that obese persons respond with inordinate strength to the appearance of food. By extrapolation it can be shown that obese persons are influenced by the appearance of the quantity of food. In a test of this notion, Stuart, as part of the unpublished study cited in Chapter 1, asked half of forty women awaiting participation in weight reduction programs to measure their food at all meals and to serve their own food on salad plates, while the other half served their measured food on dinner plates. The same amount of food on different diameter plates resulted in the differential experiences of satiety. Over 70 percent of the women reported greater satisfaction with the quantity of meals served on salad plates despite the fact that they served the portions themselves and knew them to be equal to the portions served on larger dinner plates. Therefore it is wise for a dieter to:

MAKE SMALL PORTIONS OF FOOD APPEAR TO BE AS LARGE AS POSSIBLE

either by serving on smaller plates or by spreading the food out on the surface of the plate.

SUPPRESSION STEP FIVE

As was mentioned earlier, eating leads to both positive and negative reinforcement — positive reinforcement associated with the pleasure intrinsic in the taste and smell of food as well as the actual act of eating, negative reinforcement associated with the termination of states of deprivation. While the positive reinforcement value of food can be controlled by, for example, purchasing ice cream in flavors favored by other family members but not strongly liked by the overeater, it is equally important to:

CONTROL STATES OF DEPRIVATION

There are three types of deprivation which appear to be phenomenologically linked to problematic eating. The first is food deprivation. When an overeater skips a meal he puts himself in a state of deprivation which automatically increases the positive value of food. He also appears psychologically to have become indebted to himself for additional eating and thus has a strong tendency to overeat at his next feeding. This can be avoided by the simple expedient of *planning meals for regular hours and eating every planned meal.* The second type of deprivation is "energy" deprivation. Overeaters have frequently been found to associate great amounts of overeating with times when they are fatigued, generally due to lack of sleep. Whether the natural energy store is somehow depleted by sleep deprivation or whether fatigue is a conditioned cue for eating, it is clearly essential for the overeater to *take pains to avoid fatigue due to sleep loss.* Second only in importance to attention to food intake and energy expenditure, the careful monitoring of sleep patterns is an essential element in the effective control of overeating.

The third type of deprivation commonly associated with problematic overeating is the stimulus deprivation experienced as boredom. There is good clinical evidence in support of the supposition that eating is not a preferred pastime for obese persons. In fact, the forty obese subjects questioned by Stuart in the earlier unpublished study ranked eating fifth in a hierarchy of five activities behind, in order, socializing, work and affectionate-sexual encounters (which were tied), and personal, nonfood pleasures; only two members of the entire sample ranked eating as either first or second in importance. Therefore it can be supposed that eating could be displaced by any of a number of other activities which would result in sustained attention and positive gratification. Since it appears to be important that boredom be avoided if at all possible, it is helpful for each overeater to keep available to himself at all times a number of nonfood activities capable of engaging his interest. Whether these activities are social (e.g., visiting or phoning friends), work (e.g., vocational or home business such as balancing the checkbook), or avocational (e.g., traditional hobbies or reading), a range of nonfood-related activities should be constantly available as responses to compete with eating. Furthermore, in an effort to strengthen the probability that these responses will occur in place of eating, they should be available with a minimum of effort. In the service of this objective, the sewing machine should be kept up at all times; interesting books, records, or magazines should be in clear view at all times; or gardening implements and plans should always be available depending upon the value of these or other pleasures for the overeater.

* * * * *

The five suppression steps were all designed to weaken the impact which problematic foods might have upon the behavior of an overeater. Probably the best way to weaken the impact of a problematic antecedent, however, is to displace it with a strong cue which sets the occasion for the emission of a desirable behavior. This is the process of strengthening antecedents.

STRENGTHENING STEP ONE

The most important step towards the goal of strengthening the antecedents of appropriate eating is the development of a means of providing information about appropriate food choices and the allowable amounts of these foods to be eaten. For this to be done:

PROVIDE A REASONABLE ARRAY OF ACCEPTABLE FOOD CHOICES

PROVIDE FEEDBACK ABOUT THE AMOUNT WHICH CAN BE EATEN

Provision of alternatives for eating eliminates much of the discretion in food choice which introduces room for a large margin of error. Specific prescriptive diets, at one extreme, are often not useful because there are frequent occasions when the dieter simply cannot get prescribed foods such as "three tablespoons of cottage cheese on one leaf of romaine lettuce, 4 and 4/16 inches in diameter." Lacking the prescribed food, any problematic food might be chosen in its place. At the other extreme, gross limits set upon caloric intake such as "eat a moderate amount of food" are so vague as to provide virtually no guidelines. As a middle-range alternative, diets can be offered which both provide structure to eating choices and offer sufficient flexibility to allow for a realistic assortment of choices. (Such a diet will be described fully in Chapter 5.)

Beyond having an appropriate cue pointing toward which foods to eat, it is also essential for the dieter to have a means of determining how much of each food he is allowed according to his individual diet regimen. This feedback about allowable food must be available any time and any place that eating is likely to occur, must provide a cumulative total of what has been and therefore what can be eaten, and must be both a source of information and an aid to the behavioral control of eating. The feedback system described in Chapter 5 and provided in the vinyl folder appended to the book is the best means yet found for achieving these varied purposes.

When food consumption is recorded by writing in the time that each food is selected, the dieter is cued immediately as to how much he may still eat during the day. He also can have the benefit of social monitoring as another person has only to inspect the card in order to determine whether the dieter has recorded the food which he is eating at that particular moment. Taken together, the food exchange diet and the feedback form go far toward strengthening the cues associated with desirable food selections.

STRENGTHENING STEP TWO

The second step toward strengthening the control of appropriate eating is made possible by the use of food intake records as suggested in Strengthening Step 1. To complete this step:

SAVE ALLOWABLE FOODS FROM MEALS FOR SNACKS

Snacking is a treacherous act for overeaters to start. When snacks are eaten in lieu of an upcoming dessert, there is little likelihood that the dessert will be passed up. But when snacks are allocated from the preceding meal, such as saving one slice of breakfast toast as a snack with mid-morning coffee at a prescribed time, the wish for mid-morning food can be granted without doing violence to the general eating program.

STRENGTHENING STEP THREE

As has been stated repeatedly, there is a strong indication that the eating behavior of obese persons is influenced greatly by the characteristics of the food available for their consumption. The appearance, taste, smell, and texture of the food are all important characteristics. Therefore it is important to:

MAKE ACCEPTABLE FOODS AS ATTRACTIVE AS POSSIBLE

This can be done by using low-calorie garnishments such as parsley and low-calorie embellishments such as paprika and other spices. When diet foods are pallid in contrast to less acceptable foods, the latter will be eaten. When a diet is followed there is a necessary reduction in the range of food choices, and in order to increase the acceptability of those which are eaten, it is essential to experiment with varied means of food preparation.

* * * * *

Taken together, these varied means of managing the antecedents of eating will produce an environment in which acceptable food choices are more likely to occur. It is doubtful, however, that such antecedent changes in and of themselves will result in the desired behavioral change. Therefore it is necessary to manage eating responses themselves and their consequences in an effort to modify all salient aspects of eating.

Direct management of eating responses. Many obese individuals complain of difficulty in controlling what they term as their "compulsive" eating behavior. When the eating response is given a deviance label and set aside, the individual is not encouraged to undertake changes necessary for its appropriate management. Efforts directed toward any momentary control over eating itself therefore have symbolic value above and beyond their immediate significance for the control of problematic eating.

RESPONSE STEP

The undesirable aspects of problematic eating center around the speed with which food is eaten since reductions in the pace of food consumption can significantly limit the amount eaten during the span of a normal mealtime and can slow the overeater to a pace compatible with the rate at which others eat so that he does not finish his portion well before others. Therefore it is essential to:

SLOW THE PACE OF EATING

This can be done in four ways. First, it may be helpful to *interpose a delay shortly after the start of the meal* and as frequently thereafter as may seem helpful. To do this, simply arrange to place the utensils on the plate for a predetermined time of approximately one to three minutes. The delay serves two purposes. It both gives the overeater an early experience of controlling a behavior which he had previously defined as "compulsive" and beyond his control, and also serves to slow the process of eating. Second, the pace of eating can be slowed through establishing as a rule the requirement that *food already in the mouth be swallowed before additional food is added*. One means of promoting this change is the requirement that the utensils be placed on the plate as soon as food is put in the mouth and that they not be picked up again until the food has been

89

swallowed. Third, the pace of eating can be slowed by *requiring the use of utensils at all times, and for all foods.* One can, for example, eat a sandwich far more quickly by picking it up in his hands, but eating the sandwich with a knife and fork will increase the overall time needed for its consumption. Finally, it may be helpful to resort to *counting mouthfuls per minute.* Sophisticated devices for counting chewing behavior in humans are available,[51] but simple supermarket expense counters available for less than a dollar are quite suitable for counts of mouthfuls by an individual wishing to track his own behavior. Leitenberg, Agras, and Thomson[52] have referred to the use of counts of mouthfuls as a means of increasing the eating of patients suffering from anorexia nervosa, but precisely the same procedures can be used for slowing the rate of eating by overeaters, particularly if these counts are graphed and an effort is made to gradually reduce the number of mouthfuls per minute while extending the number of minutes of the meal, holding caloric intake constant.

* * * * *

Consequences. The foregoing procedure can prove to be of great help in both partialing the strength of problematic aspects of eating and strengthening those aspects of eating which are constructive for weight management. Management of the antecedents and direct manipulation of the actual response of eating are not sufficient, however. If most human behavior is controlled by its consequences, then the consequences of problematic and effective eating must play a critical role in the control of both. It is therefore necessary to both provide decelerating consequences for problematic eating and strengthen desirable eating behaviors.

DECELERATING STEP ONE

Many people undergoing treatment for weight reduction have a similar complaint: Their overeating results in considerable attention, albeit negative, while their adherence to a dietary regimen goes unnoticed. Therefore deviations from the plan are reinforced strongly with attention while adherence undergoes extinction. It is thus essential for the social monitor to:

RESPOND NEUTRALLY TO ALL NEGATIVE DEVIATIONS FROM
A WEIGHT CONTROL PLAN

This can not only potentiate the importance of social reinforcement for adherence to the program, but it can also guard against inadvertent reinforcement of deviations. Furthermore, to the extent that eating helps to reduce tensions, the elimination of tension-producing social pressure will reduce the likelihood of stress-induced eating.

So important is it to place the major emphasis upon constructive behaviors that it is essential for professionals as well as persons in the natural environment to deal essentially with their patients' constructive response to the intervention program. To do otherwise is to risk maintenance of negative behavior by virtue of the therapist's differential attention to negative as opposed to positive behavior. When therapists are faced with the necessity of dealing with failures to follow through with a program, it is far better to arrange for discussion of how the patient might have succeeded in preference to speculating about reasons for his failure, since the former cues appropriate behavior while the latter reinforces inappropriate responses.

DECELERATING STEP TWO

In the forerunner of the present program, Ferster and his associates[53] stressed to their patients the importance of the ultimate and immediate aversive consequences of obesity. Therefore in response to overeating it may be helpful to:

BRING INTO FOCUS THE ULTIMATE AND IMMEDIATE AVERSIVE CONSEQUENCES OF OVEREATING

The ultimate consequences are the well-known heightened risk of contracting serious and incapacitating illnesses and premature death, while the immediate aversive consequences are the embarrassment, immobility, and stigmatization commonly suffered by obese individuals in this society. There is some evidence, as reflected in the decrease in smoking in the general population, that awareness of the physical consequences of a voluntary behavior may lead to its reduction although the research literature indicates that, among other things, it is important to individualize the threat and provide clear links between the present and future.[54]

* * * * *

While the deceleration of problematic responses may offer some benefit to the weight reducer, he is more likely to benefit from efforts to accelerate constructive eating. The assortment of techniques available for the acceleration of these responses draws heavily upon the major elements of feedback and altered social interaction which have gone into the program up to this point.

ACCELERATING STEP ONE

The first accelerating consequence is the provision of feedback about the rate of eating control, energy expenditure, and weight loss. While Penick and his associates believe that weight should be taken at weekly intervals to overcome the disillusionment associated with normal fluctuations in weight,[55] many obese individuals prefer to have more immediate feedback about their efforts and the results which they produce. The more immediate the feedback can be, the more powerful it is likely to be. Therefore it is necessary to:

UPDATE EATING, EXERCISE, AND WEIGHT-CHANGE GRAPHS DAILY

A form suitable for such graphing is presented in Figure 5 and can easily be reproduced on any standard-size graph paper having four or five squares per inch. While the monochromatic figure uses different types of lines, different colors for eating, exercise, and weight would probably provide more distinctive representations. Placement of the graph in a conspicuous location such as the refrigerator door can extend its usefulness from a consequence of eating to something with cue value as well, for it can cue the weight-reducer when to eat and it can alert significant others as to the appropriate times to offer social reinforcement.

Beyond familiar graphing procedures, Penick and his associates devised an ingenious means of providing feedback about weight loss. [56] They asked their patients to place in the refrigerator fifteen or twenty pieces of suet. For each pound lost they suggested that their patients remove one piece of suet as a symbol of fat loss. This is a clever way of enhancing the cue and reinforcement value of feedback about success of efforts to lose weight.

ACCELERATING STEP TWO

While social reinforcement is an important and powerful means of controlling human behavior, material consequences are at times as important or even more important. Material reinforcers have an intrinsic power with regard to mediating the occurrence of other desired events. For example, a pretty new dress is both an intrinsically reinforcing stimulus and a means of gaining social reinforcement in the form of attention, praise, or admiration. The process of delivering material reinforcers adds to their value as they set the occasion for social interchanges and they serve as unambiguous indices of positive evaluation. Therefore it is important to:

FIGURE 5

DAILY EATING, EXERCISE, AND WEIGHT GRAPH

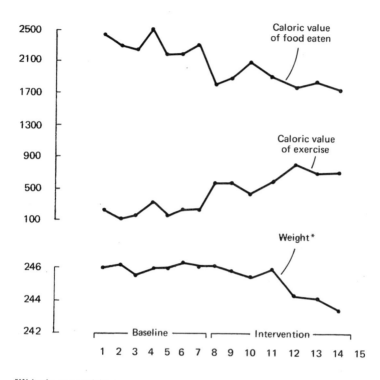

*Write in own weight range

ARRANGE FOR THE PROVISION OF MATERIAL REINFORCE-
MENT FOLLOWING COMPLETION OF EATING AND EXERCISE
REQUIREMENTS AND/OR WEIGHT LOSS

For many years people were well aware of the value of material
consequences in promoting high rates of human and animal behavior, but
there was always difficulty in using material reinforcers because to be
useful they had to be in fairly large units. Some five millenia ago, however,
man began to use some form of token as a medium of exchange which
enabled him to symbolically transfer the equivalent of the hind quarter of
a deer for two good women and enough grain to bake forty loaves of
bread. This system evolved into the monetary system with which we are
quite familiar and then into the use of tokens as a means of controlling the
behavior of people in many environments where the use of money as a
reinforcer is impractical.[57] Applied to weight control programs, tokens

can be given on the basis of adherence to caloric restrictions each mealtime or each day, completion of differing amounts of energy expenditure, or achievement of weight-loss objectives on a daily or weekly basis. In general, the smaller the unit of behavior the better, because small behavioral units occur frequently and provide an opportunity for frequent positive feedback and reinforcing experiences. Beyond the social value of tokens, it is often helpful to attach a material value as reflected in a "menu" for token redemptions. A sample menu linking responses and reinforcers is illustrated in Figure 6. Items can be valued or added to the menu according to individual preferences, and the gaming aspect of the token system can be played up or down as suits the style of the person or persons seeking to lose weight. The important point is that token consequences must be provided immediately following the response and must be exchangeable for items valued by the behaver. Finally, it should be noted that whether or not tokens or other material reinforcements are offered as consequences for weight change, it is always essential to offer tokens for each act of compliance with a weight management program. This requirement stems from the fact that the payoff of compliance as measured by weight loss may be somewhat delayed, and it is essential to provide mediating reinforcements which will maintain the very active steps needed to produce weight loss.

FIGURE 6
TOKEN REINFORCEMENT MENU

Responses Earning Tokens		
Response	Amount	No. Tokens
Follow diet	1 meal	3
Follow diet	3 consecutive meals	12
Follow diet	7 consecutive days	100
Walk	1 block	.5
Walk	6 blocks	6
Walk	20 blocks	25

Redemption Value of Tokens	
Item	No. Tokens
Extra 15 min. conversation	3
Extra evening out	25
Extra baby sitter for 3 hours during day	25
$2 surprise	300
New dress	500
Special weekend trip	1500

ACCELERATING STEP THREE

Feedback about compliance with a weight management program and material reinforcement for each successful effort are important accelerating consequences which in and of themselves may positively influence behavior. The strength of each, however, can be increased through the addition of social reinforcement. Therefore it is important for the social monitor to:

PROVIDE SOCIAL REINFORCEMENT FOR ALL CONSTRUCTIVE EFFORTS TO MODIFY WEIGHT-RELEVANT BEHAVIORS

Some of these efforts will pertain directly to weight loss, others to general attitudes about food and energy expenditures. It is important for the weight-reducer to discuss his activities only with those who are likely to be sympathetic toward his objectives, and it is important for those with whom these activities are discussed to provide as much encouragement and as little questioning as possible. This is in keeping with the general requirement that an effective weight-control program must lead to a general reorganization of the role of energy intake and output in the life of an individual, and broad changes of this character are likely to be reflected in general philosophical beliefs about what constitutes the "good life." For the person effectively controlling his weight, the good life must be expanded to include intelligent decisions with respect to the energy balance and must be narrowed to exclude the pursuit of opportunities to overeat and underexercise.

Conclusion. A program leading to weight reduction has been described from the point of view of the situational versus the self-control aspects of food intake and energy expenditure. The program is based upon efforts to manipulate antecedent, response, and consequent variables in a manner conducive to specific behavioral changes. Whether the changes are effective is a matter for individual determination. The various steps suggested are illustrative of the techniques used successfully with an all-female experimental sample over 200 strong. In each instance it was found expedient to *individualize specific procedures* within the rubric of a general approach to situational management. When the overeater lives with others, whether family members or roommates, it has proven essential to *include* significant others in the initial planning and execution of the program. These others are a source of information about relevant environmental conditions of which the overeater himself may be unaware as well as crucial allies in the weight-reducing process. In the unpublished study by Stuart frequently alluded to above, the cooperation of these other persons proved critical with respect to treatment outcome. Eighty-three percent of those subjects who could name and work with another person to aid in cueing and reinforcing appropriate eating lost 20 percent or more of body weight and maintained this loss for at least a 12-month post-treatment follow-up. Only 31 percent of those who did not have the cooperation of at least one other person met with this same degree of success. These results should clearly illustrate the crucial role to be played by other people in what is essentially a general process involving the social control of problematic behavior.

Beyond these qualifications, other minor suggestions have come from clinical experience with this program. It is wise, for example, *not to undertake a weight control program shortly before a holiday.* That is, it is not likely that an intervention program will be effective when opposed by massive and concentrated social pressure to eat excessively. Such an early failure can preclude the possibility of any eventual enthusiasm for the program. Second, it has been found helpful to *make clear at the outset that a weight-control program may lead to new and unanticipated expenses.* As significant amounts of weight are lost, clothing expenses rise. Because of this it is wise to defer clothing purchases whenever a weight reduction program is begun and to wear tatters and rags if need be until target weights are achieved. This, incidentally, adds an additional material incentive to weight control while helping to offset the cost of weight reduction. Finally, it has been learned that an effective program is one which *plans for occasional reintroduction to specific situational changes,* such as the reinstigation of social monitoring, as a means of maintaining weight changes. Maintenance is the "stepchild" of most behavior control programs which, if overlooked, can lead to the gradual dissipation of any and all constructive changes. In this vein it is probably wise to continue the monitoring of both energy intake and output continuously until appropriate controls become "wired in" or automatic, even then returning to objective monitoring periodically.

FOOTNOTES

1. Gordon, E. S. The present concept of obesity: Etiological factors and treatment. *Medical Times*, 1969, *97*, 148.
2. Stunkard, A. and McLaren-Hume, M. The results of treatment for obesity. *Archives of Internal Medicine*, 1959, *103*, 79-85.
3. Penick, S. B., Filion, R., Fox, S., and Stunkard, A. J. Behavior modification treatment of obesity. Paper presented at the annual meeting of the American Psychosomatic Society, Washington, D.C., March 1970.
4. Mayer, J. Genetic, traumatic and environmental factors in the etiology of obesity. *Physiological Review*, 1953, *33*, 472-508.
5. Azrin, N.H. and Powell, J. Behavioral engineering: The reduction of smoking behavior by a conditioning apparatus and procedure. *Journal of Applied Behavior Analysis*, 1968, *1*, 193-200.
6. Stuart, R. B. Operant interpersonal treatment of marital discord. *Journal of Consulting and Clinical Psychology*, 1969, *33*, 675-682; and Byrne, D. and Rhamey, R. Magnitude of positive and negative reinforcements as a determinant of attraction. *Journal of Personality and Social Psychology*, 1965, *2*, 884-889.
7. Azrin, N. H. and Holz, W. C. Punishment. In W. R. Honig (Ed.), *Operant behavior: Areas of research and application.* New York: Appleton-Century-Crofts, 1966.
8. Bucher, B. and Lovaas, O.I. Operant procedures in behavior modification with children. In D. J. Levis (Ed.), *Learning approaches to therapeutic behavior change.* Chicago: Aldine, 1970.
9. Moss, F. A. Note on building likes and dislikes in children. *Journal of Experimental Psychology*, 1924, *7*, 475-478.
10. Wolpe, J. Reciprocal inhibition as the main basis of psychotherapeutic effects. *Archives of Neurology and Psychiatry*, 1954, *72*, 205-226.
11. Meyer, V. and Crisp, A. H. Aversion therapy in two cases of obesity. *Behaviour Research and Therapy*, 1964, *2*, 143-147.
12. Stollak, G. E. Weight loss obtained under different experimental procedures. *Psychotherapy, Theory, Research and Practice*, 1967, *4*, 51-64.
13. Kennedy, W. A. and Foreyt, J. P. Control of eating behavior in an obese patient by avoidance conditioning. *Psychological Reports*, 1968, *22*, 571-576.
14. Cautela, J. R. Treatment of compulsive behavior by covert sensitization. *Psychological Record*, 1966, *16*, 33-41.
15. *Ibid.;* and Stuart, R. B. Behavioral control of overeating. *Behaviour Research and Therapy*, 1967, *5*, 357-365.
16. Tyler, V. O. and Straughan, J. H. Coverant control and breath holding as techniques for the treatment of obesity. *Psychological Record*, 1970, *20*, 473-478.
17. *Ibid.*
18. Homme, L. E. Perspectives in psychology: XXIV. Control of coverants, the operants of the mind. *Psychological Record*, 1965, *15*, 501-511.
19. Horan, J. J. The effect of coverant conditioning on weight reduction. Paper presented at the annual meeting of the American Educational Research Association, 1971.
20. For example, see Andelman, M. B., Jones, C., and Nathan, S. Treatment of obesity in underprivileged adolescents. *Clinical Pediatrics*, 1967, *6*, 327-330; and Young, C.M., Moore, N.S., Beresford, K., Einset, B.M., and Waldner, B.G. The problem of the obese patient, *Journal of the American Dietetic Association*, 1955, *3*, 1111-1115.
21. Cautela, *op. cit.*; and Stuart, Behavioral control, *op. cit.*
22. Ferster, C. B., Nurnberger, J. L., and Levitt, E. B. The control of eating. *Journal of Mathetics*, 1962, *1*, 87-109.
23. Stuart, Behavioral control, *op. cit.*
24. Harris, M. B. Self-directed program for weight control: A pilot study. *Journal of Abnormal Psychology*, 1969, *74*, 263-270.
25. *Ibid.*, p. 265.
26. Wollersheim, J. P. Effectiveness of group therapy based upon learning principles in the treatment of overweight women. *Journal of Abnormal Psychology*, 1970, *76*, 462-474.

27. See Stunkard, A., Levine, H., and Fox, S. The management of obesity. *Archives of Internal Medicine*, 1970, *125*, 1067-1072; Kornhaber, A. Group treatment of obesity. *GP*, 1968, *38*, 116-120; and Wagonfeld, S. and Wolowitz, H. M. Obesity and the self-help group: A look at TOPS. *American Journal of Psychiatry*, 1968, *125*, 253-255.
28. Rosenthal, R. *Experimenter effects in behavioral research.* New York: Appleton-Century-Crofts, 1966.
29. Penick *et al., op. cit.*
30. Ayllon, T. Intensive treatment of psychotic behaviour by stimulus satiation and food reinforcement. *Behaviour Research and Therapy*, 1963, *1*, 53-61.
31. Harmatz, M. G. and Lapuc, P. Behavior modification of overeating in a psychiatric population. *Journal of Consulting and Clinical Psychology*, 1968, *32*, 583-587.
32. Barnard, J.L. Rapid treatment of gross obesity by operant techniques. *Psychological Reports*, 1968, *23*, 663-668.
33. Mann, R. A. The behavior-therapeutic use of contingency contracting to control adult behavior problems: Weight control. *Journal of Applied Behavior Analysis*, in press.
34. Stuart, R. B. Behavioral contracting within the families of delinquents. *Journal of Behaviour Therapy and Experimental Psychiatry*, 1971, *2*, 1-11.
35. Stuart, Behavioral control, *op. cit.*
36. Penick *et al., op. cit.*
37. Stuart, Behavioral control, *op. cit.*
38. Harris, *op. cit.*, p. 268.
39. Wollersheim, *op. cit.*
40. Stunkard, A. J. The dieting depression. *American Journal of Medicine*, 1957, *12*, 77-86.
41. Penick *et al., op. cit.*
42. Wollersheim, *op. cit.*
43. Harris, *op. cit.*
44. Penick *et al., op. cit.*
45. Nisbett, R. E. and Kanouse, D. E. Obesity, food deprivation, and supermarket shopping behavior. *Journal of Personality and Social Psychology*, 1969, *12*, 289-294.
46. Gordon, *op. cit.*
47. For example, see Debry, G., Rohr, R., Azouaou, G., Vassilitch, I., and Mottaz, G. Study of the effect of dividing the daily caloric intake into seven meals on weight loss in obese subjects. *Nutritio et Dieta*, 1968, *10*, 288-296.
48. Patterson, G. R., Hawkins, N., McNeal, S., and Phelps, R. Reprogramming the social environment. *Journal of Child Psychology and Psychiatry*, 1967, *8*, 181-196.
49. Stuart, R. B. A critical reappraisal and reformulation of selected mental health problems. In L. A. Hamerlynck, P. O. Davidson, and L. E. Acker (Eds.), *Behavior modification and ideal mental health services.* Calgary: University of Calgary Press, 1969.
50. Mayer, *op. cit.*
51. Rugh, J. D. A telemetry system for measuring chewing behavior in humans. *Behavior Research Methods and Instruments*, 1971, *3*, 73-77.
52. Leitenberg, H., Agras, W. S., and Thomson, L. E. A sequential analysis of the effect of selective positive reinforcement in modifying anorexia nervosa. *Behaviour Research and Therapy*, 1968, *6*, 211-218.
53. Ferster *et al., op. cit.*
54. Leventhal, H. Fear communications in the acceptance of preventive health practices. *Bulletin of the New York Academy of Medicine*, 1965, *41*, 1144-1168.
55. Penick *et al., op. cit.*
56. *Ibid.*
57. Ayllon, T., and Azrin, N. H. *The token economy.* New York: Appleton-Century-Crofts, 1968.

Chapter 4
NUTRITION

Man instinctively eats food to relieve the uncomfortable symptoms of hunger. He does not, however, instinctively choose the foods that fulfill all his physiological needs and result in optimum health. Early man probably consumed a wide variety of foods, learning through trial and sometimes disastrous error which were beneficial and which were not. Although always preoccupied with food, it is only in the past century, with the development of nutritional science, that man has learned what food does for him and what his nutritional needs are. Today however, as in the past, availability of food, social and cultural influences, and personal preferences often affect his choices to a greater extent than the desire for a nutritious diet.

NUTRITION IN THE AFFLUENT SOCIETY

It might be supposed that in educated affluent societies the selection of a nutritious diet would not be a problem. In the United States, however, suspicions are being aroused that the population is not as well-nourished as was previously believed. The major nutritional problem for many Americans is neither a scarcity of food nor the severe lack of a specific food or food ingredients, but rather the consumption of more food than needed, resulting in excessive fat storage and obesity.[1] The facts and figures on the prevalence of obesity and its relationship to health, discussed in Chapter 1, strengthen the suggestion that changes are needed in the eating practices of many Americans. In today's society it is probably more important to train children to recognize when they have had sufficient amounts of food than to stress the necessity of a "clean plate," as prevention rather than cure is perhaps the simplest solution for the condition.

Furthermore, many people are choosing diets overbalanced in foods containing high concentrations of sugars and animal fats,[2] and they thereby neglect foods containing other needed ingredients. One panel at the recent White House Conference on Food, Nutrition, and Health concluded that the affluent society is characterized by:

1. Overconsumption of calories with food choices that are not necessarily the wisest on the basis of available nutritional information; [and]

2. Underexercising and failure to develop life-long habits to combat the ills of a sedentary life.[3]

The results of the 1965 survey made by the United States Department of Agriculture on a representative sample of the population supports the viewpoint that Americans are not choosing their foods wisely.[4] This survey indicated that only 50 percent of the households surveyed had diets which were rated as "good," that is, which met the United States Recommended Daily Allowances for the seven nutrients evaluated — protein, calcium, iron, vitamins A and C, thiamine, and riboflavin. This represented a decrease in quality from a 1955 survey (see Figure 1). Calcium and iron were the nutrients most frequently found lacking overall, however in the lowest income class and for persons in the Southern regions, vitamins A and C were most often below the recommended allowances.

FIGURE 1
QUALITY OF DIETS
1955 — 1965

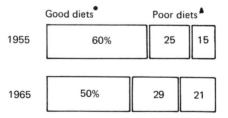

•Met recommended dietary allowances (1964) for 7 nutrients
▲Had less than 2/3 allowance for 1 to 7 nutrients
Nationwide Household Food Consumption Survey Spring 1955 and Spring 1965

Reproduced with permission from S. F. Adelson, Changes in diets of households, 1955 to 1965. *Journal of Home Economics,* 1968, *60,* 451.

FIGURE 2
INCOME AND QUALITY OF DIETS

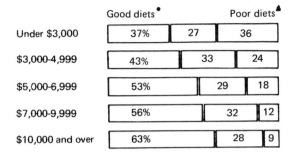

●Met recommended dietary allowances for 7 nutrients
▲Had less than 2/3 allowance for 1 to 7 nutrients
Nationwide Household Food Consumption Survey Spring 1965

Reproduced with permission from S. F. Adelson, Changes in diets of households, 1955 to 1965. *Journal of Home Economics*, 1968, 60, 450.

A review article comparing findings of the 1965 study with that of 1955 reported:

> Despite higher income and the opportunity to choose from the greatest abundance of foods in the U.S. history, there has been a somewhat adverse shift in household food consumption and thus in dietary levels in the past decade.[5]

Quality of the diets was directly related to income. However, poor diets occurred at even the highest income levels (see Figure 2). Thus although for the poor of America there exists a scarcity of food,[6] for the majority of people the problem is to choose a balanced diet from an overwhelming selection of foods. Because investigations indicate that many Americans are not choosing such a diet, can it be assumed that the health of the population is being adversely affected?

The deficiency diseases that traditionally characterize malnourished individuals are rare in America. Retarded growth patterns are also a sign of poor nutrition, yet American children are, in general, taller and heavier than their parents. For example, elementary school children in Philadelphia were on the average three inches taller and 3 pounds heavier in 1951 than in 1925.[7] Americans, then, do not seem to be exhibiting overt clinical signs of malnourishment. Thus it is to the more subtle long-term effects that scientists are turning in order to evaluate the effect on health of the typical American diet.

The influence of diet on cardiovascular diseases such as athero-

FIGURE 3
FACTORS SUSPECTED TO INFLUENCE THE
DEVELOPMENT OF ATHEROSCLEROSIS

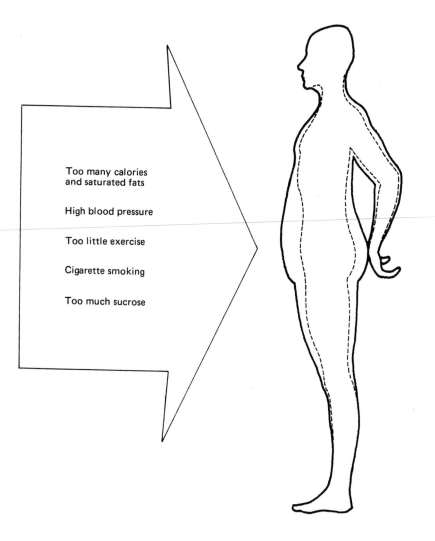

Too many calories
and saturated fats

High blood pressure

Too little exercise

Cigarette smoking

Too much sucrose

Adapted from W. B. Kannel, The disease of living, *Nutrition Today,* 1971,
6,(3), 2-11.

sclerosis and its sequela coronary heart disease is currently being investigated. Not only are such diseases a leading cause of death in the United States and their prevalence increasing, but they are striking men at an earlier age. Present statistics[8] indicate that the average healthy American man has one chance in five of suffering a heart attack before age 65, and furthermore, that only one man in five survives such an attack. Women appear to have some protection, at least until the menopause, as three times as many men as women succumb to heart disease.[9] However, both American men and women are twice as likely to die of a fatal heart attack as Norwegian, Swedish, and Dutch men and women.[10] Exhaustive research into the etiology of atherosclerosis implicates a combination of factors including the high-calorie diet rich in sugars and animal fats commonly consumed by many Americans (see Figure 3).[11] Preventive measures are necessary for these critical diseases, and it is generally felt that changes in eating habits early in life are an essential part of prophylactic measures.

Another area where diet may have an effect is in the outcome of pregnancy. In 1967 the infant mortality rate in the United States reached a record high of 22.4 deaths per 1,000 live births and ranked poorer than 12 other industrialized nations in this respect.[12] While it is difficult to separate the effects of nutrition from other factors, Dr. Robert E. Shank, Chairman of the Committee on Maternal Nutrition of the Food and Nutrition Board of the National Research Council, has cited poor nutrition and youth of the mother as among the factors contributing to poor pregnancy outcome.[13] A summary of the findings of this committee stated:

> Nutrition has an important role in reproductive performance. Epidemiological data strongly suggest that good preparation for pregnancy is based on good health background and good nutritional status. To be well nourished from childhood and to maintain good diet during pregnancy would help to ensure safe, healthy pregnancies and healthy babies.[14]

Other aspects of health, such as the ability to resist or recover readily from infections,[15] are undoubtedly affected by diet; however, it is extremely difficult to separate the influence of diet from other factors such as genetic determinants, physical exercise, and environmental and psychological stresses. Common sense indicates that optimum functioning of the human body must be strongly affected by the raw materials supplied to it and that good nutrition contributes to the vitality, emotional stability, and general appearance of the healthy individual.[16]

The current concern with the typical American diet has aroused interest in the subject of diet and nutrition, as reflected by the numerous articles in the popular press. The conventional approach when supplying nutritional information is to discuss individual food nutrients and the clinical symptoms resulting from a lack of each. It has been decided instead to focus this chapter on the biochemical functions of nutrients within the body as well as the place the various nutrients occupy in the typical American diet.

THE NUTRIENTS

The human body has the amazing capacity to synthesize thousands of chemical compounds needed for its complex and intricate metabolic processes. Forty or so of these compounds — called nutrients — serve either as raw materials or as catalytic agents for these processes and must be supplied by food. Table 1 lists the nutrients known to play an essential role in the growth and maintenance of the body. This list is perhaps not complete for a number of reasons. First, there are minerals such as flourine which seem to be beneficial, but it has not been determined whether they are essential. In addition there are certain vitamin-like substances needed

TABLE 1

LIST OF NUTRIENTS

Carbohydrate
  Glucose

Fat or lipid
  Linoleic acid

Protein
  Amino acids
    Leucine
    Isoleucine
    Lysine
    Methionine
    Phenylalanine
    Threonine
    Trytophan
    Valine
  Nonessential nitrogen

Minerals
  Calcium
  Phosphorus
  Sodium
  Potassium
  Sulphur
  Chlorine
  Magnesium
  Iron
  Selenium

Zinc
Manganese
Copper
Cobalt
Molybdenum
Iodine
Chromium
Fluorine

Vitamins
  Fat-soluble vitamins
    A
    D
    E
    K
  Water-soluble vitamins
    Thiamine
    Riboflavin
    Niacin
    Biotin
    Folacin
    Pyridoxine
    Cobalamin
    Pantothenic acid
    Ascorbic acid

Water

Reproduced with permission from H. A. Guthrie, *Introductory Nutrition* (2nd ed.). St. Louis, Mo.: C. V. Mosby, 1971. P. 10.

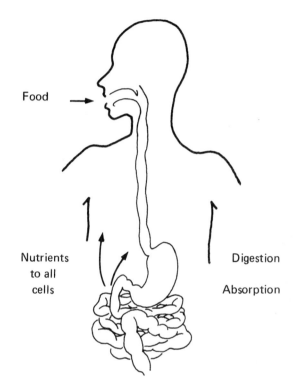

Food

Nutrients
to all
cells

Digestion

Absorption

for normal metabolism which the body can synthesize, but additional sources may have to be supplied in the diet which would classify them as nutrients. Finally, it is always possible that there are unknown constituents of foods that are needed in trace amounts. Until all the metabolic mysteries of the body have been defined, the list of nutrients will likely not be completed.

Nutrients are released from food through the action of the digestive system. They are then absorbed, some are altered chemically, and all are transported via the blood to the body cells (see Figure 4). Each cell is surrounded by a fluid of nutrients and it selects and uses what it needs in order to perform its own specific task. Cellular work is accomplished through myriads of intricate step-by-step chemical reactions taking place on the nutrients, either breaking them down to release their trapped energy or transforming and combining them to form new materials.

Countless chemical reactions occur simultaneously within the cells, and metabolism is the term used to cover the entire process. These basic biochemical processes of energy production and growth taking place within the living cell are the same or very similar in all cells — whether cells of the human body, of other animals, of plants, or of microorganisms. The discovery of this "unity of biochemistry" has been one of the most exciting scientific achievements of the century.[17]

Whereas the one-celled organism exists in direct contact with its environment, selecting its needed nutrients for energy and cell maintenance from this environment and excreting waste materials directly into it, multicelled organisms have had to develop complex systems in order to satisfy cellular needs. Cells performing similar kinds of work form tissue; several types of tissue are combined to form organs having specific functions; and organs are arranged into systems. Each system performs a specific role but all are integrated to result in the efficient functioning of the human body. Perfect or optimal nutrition may be defined as the state where every cell is constantly supplied with the nutrients it needs when they are needed. It is impossible, however, to assess the nutritional needs of every cell.

Estimates of Nutrient Needs. While it is impossible to determine cellular needs, scientists are able to estimate the amounts of nutrients needed to prevent clinical signs of nutritional deficiencies. Suggested amounts are based on these estimates plus an added safety allowance. In the United States, the Food and Nutrition Board of the National Research Council, National Academy of Sciences, has developed a table of Recommended Dietary Allowances (RDA) which are periodically revised as knowledge of nutritional needs expands (see Appendix B). These allowances consider the fact that normal individuals vary considerably in their nutritional requirements and thus are intended to cover the needs of not only the average individual but of all healthy individuals in the population. Although some forty nutrients are known to be essential, the Recommended Dietary Allowances of 1968 lists recommended amounts for but sixteen of these as well as estimations of calorie requirements. There are several reasons for this. The human requirement for many nutrients cannot as yet be well-defined, while for other nutrients, deficiencies or excesses do not appear to occur in man. However it is generally believed that if a diet provides the nutrient recommendations established by the RDA, then other nutrient needs will be satisfied.

A second set of dietary allowances, called the Minimum Daily Requirements (MDR), is used by the Food and Drug Administration as standards for the food industries when labeling the nutrient content of their products. They are based on the amounts of nutrients required to prevent deficiency disease and are generally lower than the RDA's. The existence of two sets of standards is confusing; however, in this book the Recommended Dietary Allowances will be used for they are directed towards optimal health rather than merely disease prevention.

Nutrient Groups and Their Roles in the Human Body. *Energy.* While the energy supplied in food cannot be officially classed as a nutrient, it is nevertheless the main nutritional requirement of the human body. All three major components of food — fats, carbohydrates, and proteins — may be metabolized within the body to release energy. In most diets, carbohydrates and fats are the main sources of energy thus allowing protein to be used for the synthesis and maintenance of body tissue. When food energy is lacking, the body will consume its fat stores, its dietary protein, and eventually its own tissue in order to satisfy its energy needs.

The chemical processes producing this energy are the same in all cells and can be compared to the burning of a fire. Just as fuel is oxidized or burned to produce energy and by-products, in each body cell step-by-step chemical reactions methodically break down large nutrient molecules which are oxidized to release small packets of chemical energy (see Figure 5). The amount of energy produced is measured in units of kilocalories; however, when referring to food energy this term is generally shortened to calories. When fat is the source of fuel, more than twice as many calories are provided as when either protein or carbohydrates are used (see Table 2).

FIGURE 5
DIAGRAMMATIC REPRESENTATION OF
CELLULAR OXIDATION

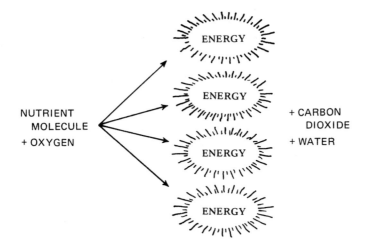

TABLE 2

ENERGY VALUES OF THE THREE ENERGY
PRODUCING NUTRIENTS IN FOODS

Nutrient	Available energy in calories per gram
Fat	9.0
Carbohydrate	4.0
Protein	4.0

The Recommended Dietary Allowances specify the caloric allowance for varying ages and for both sexes (see Appendix B). Energy needs, however, vary considerably with different levels of physical activity.

Protein. The major structural component of animal cells is protein. All forms of life, from microscopic to man, have their own characteristic proteins, yet all proteins are formed from the same twenty or so relatively simple chemical compounds called amino acids. These amino acids are strung together like links on a chain and then wound into various shapes and configurations (see Figure 6). It is the number and arrangement of

FIGURE 6

DIAGRAMMATIC REPRESENTATION OF THE WAY
AMINO ACIDS LINK UP TO FORM PROTEINS

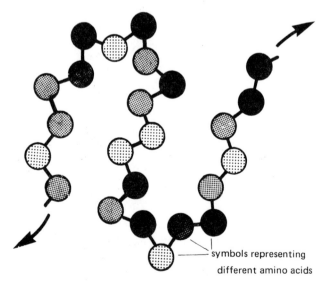

symbols representing
different amino acids

FIGURE 7

**DIAGRAMMATIC REPRESENTATION OF AMINO ACIDS
FROM FOOD PROTEIN CONVERTED TO BODY PROTEIN**

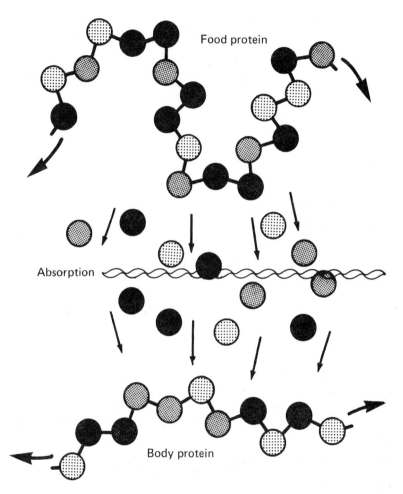

Food protein

Absorption

Body protein

these links and the shape of the resulting protein molecule that form a specific protein. The pattern to form these differences is contained in the genetic material of every cell, thus each animal species forms proteins characteristic of itself, and within a species the protein of each animal is unique.

The digestive processes break proteins down into their amino acid components, which are absorbed and transported to the cells where they are recombined and built, according to the genetic directions, into new and needed body proteins (see Figure 7). These protein molecules are very

FIGURE 8
METABOLIC FUNCTIONS OF PROTEINS

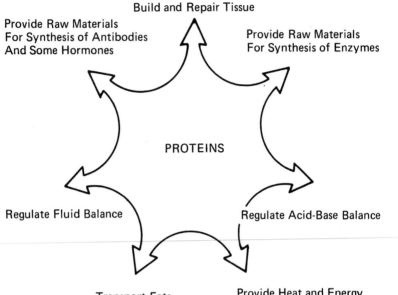

large and may contain hundreds of individual amino acids. Just as an alphabet of twenty-six letters can form a seemingly endless variety of words, so may twenty amino acids form an infinitely large number of proteins. The hemoglobin molecule represents an example of the specificity of proteins. This molecule, with its four chains of amino acids, carries needed oxygen to all the body cells. Change but one amino acid in a chain and the molecule no longer functions efficiently, resulting in the disease sickle cell anemia.

As well as forming a structural part of every living cell, special protein molecules, called enzymes, are needed to catalyze and control all metabolic reactions. The synthesis of these enzymes is also directed by the cellular genetic pattern. They are the major protein components of the cell, and there may be as many as a thousand within each cell. Many enzymes are specific for only one chemical reaction, while others are more general and can be used to direct several reactions. If an organism lacks but one crucial enzyme, this metabolic error may lead to disease or even death.

In man proteins serve other purposes as well as these two crucial ones of cellular structure and enzyme synthesis. As mentioned earlier, proteins may also be used for energy if calories from fats and carbohydrates are insufficient, and in fact, energy needs take precedence over those of growth. The multiple roles of proteins are illustrated in Figure 8.

The body has limited powers to convert one amino acid into another However there are eight, called essential amino acids, that cannot be built from others and therefore must be supplied in the diet. These are listed in Table 1. From these eight, when supplied in sufficient amounts, the remaining amino acids can be synthesized. Proteins containing these eight

FIGURE 9
PROTEIN CONTENT OF SOME TYPICAL FOODS

% Protein

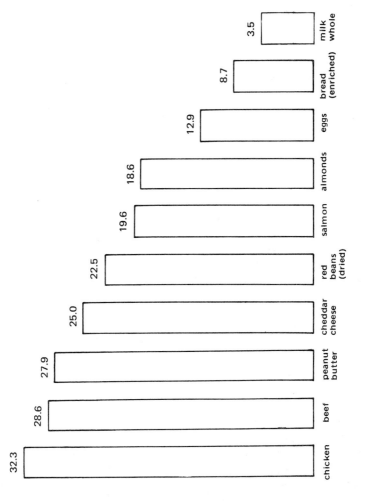

amino acids in generous amounts are said to be good-quality protein. Animal proteins have an amino acid composition similar to human proteins and therefore are good sources of the essential amino acids. Plant proteins differ more from human proteins in their amino acid composition and provide lesser amounts of some of the essential amino acids. However different plants, when combined or supplemented with small amounts of animal protein, may complement each other in amino acid composition and provide adequate amounts of the essential amino acids.

It is frequently argued that protein beyond the amounts estimated for growth and maintenance is beneficial, however this has not been proven scientifically.[18] Dietary surveys indicate that Americans do consume protein above the recommended allowance;[19] therefore most Americans, particularly adults, probably satisfy their protein requirements.[20] It must be pointed out, though, that many animal products supply plentiful amounts of fat, and in sedentary populations excessive consumption of these foods can lead to obesity and perhaps other health problems.

The table of Recommended Dietary Allowances specifies the protein allowances for both sexes and for different age levels (see Appendix B). Children have greater protein needs than adults due to the demands of growth, hence it is children who suffer most when dietary sources of

FIGURE 10
METABOLIC FUNCTIONS OF CARBOHYDRATES

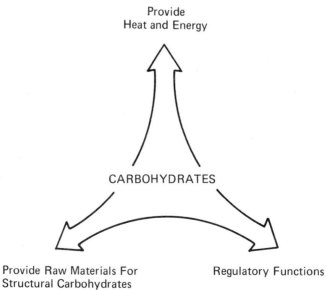

Provide
Heat and Energy

CARBOHYDRATES

Provide Raw Materials For
Structural Carbohydrates

Regulatory Functions

protein are sparse. Protein needs are also increased during pregnancy and lactation. Figure 9 shows the protein content of some commonly eaten foods.

Carbohydrates. The major physiological role of carbohydrates is to produce the energy needed for body work. In fact, in most societies, it is the carbohydrate-rich foods which make the greatest contribution toward satisfying the energy requirements of the human body. Along with this major function, carbohydrates play other minor, but necessary, roles. Some are used to form a structural component of certain body compounds while others are needed to help regulate normal metabolic functions (see Figure 10).

FIGURE 11
CHANGING PATTERNS IN CARBOHYDRATE CONSUMPTION SINCE 1889

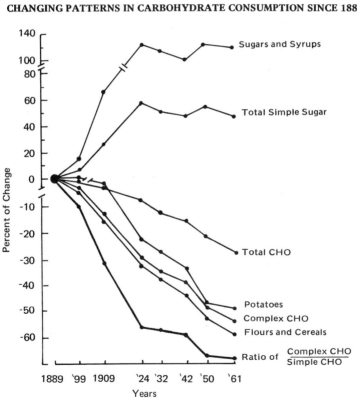

Reproduced with permission from M.A. Antar, M. A. Ohlson, and R. E. Hodges, Changes in retail market food supplies in the United States in the last seventy years in relation to the incidence of coronary heart disease, with special reference to dietary carbohydrates and essential fatty acids. *American Journal of Clinical Nutrition*, 1964, *14*, 169.

Two types of carbohydrates, starches and sugars, are broken down by the digestive processes into small soluble molecules that can be absorbed into the blood stream and transported to the cells. The simple chemical substance glucose is the predominant product of these digestive processes. Chemical reactions within the cells release the energy stored in the glucose molecule so it can be used for work and heat. As glucose can be formed from some amino acids, it has been suggested by some researchers that carbohydrates are not a dietary essential.[21] Other studies, however, report deleterious effects from diets lacking carbohydrates.[22] It is generally concluded that for many physiological reasons it is wise to include some carbohydrates in all diets[23] including those designed for weight control.[24]

Man has traditionally relied on the starches of grains and root vegetables for his main sources of carbohydrates, and the sugar sucrose is a comparative newcomer in his diet. Its flavor is appealing to man and sugar consumption has risen enormously in the past 100 years (see Figure 11), however there are indications that a high sugar intake is not compatible with optimum health. Sugars and sweets are commonly known to be associated with tooth decay.[25] A high concentration of sucrose in the diet is also suspected to influence glucose tolerance and some types of diabetes.[26] Furthermore, some research indicates that high concentrations of sugar may be a factor in the etiology of the disease atherosclerosis.[27] Finally, it must be pointed out that man's fondness for sweets encourages him to overeat and these excesses are converted to fat, contributing to the obese state. For all these reasons, individuals might consider reducing their sugar intake and using it as an occasional flavoring substance rather than a major source of energy.

The Recommended Dietary Allowances has not recommended a specific allowance for carbohydrates, however in the average American diet carbohydrates provide about 45 to 55 percent of the total calories[28] and a lack of this nutrient is not a problem. Figure 12 illustrates the carbohydrate content of some typical foods.

Fats. Fats are composed of long chains of chemical compounds called fatty acids which are chemically bonded to a molecule of the alcohol glycerol. The digestive processes break down these complex fats into simpler substances that can be absorbed through the digestive tract, transported to cells, and then either used to yield energy or recombined into fat for storage. A certain proportion of stored fat is essential, for it not only acts as an energy reserve during times of stress but helps insulate the body from the effects of the environment. Fat deposits surrounding the vital organs, for example, help to prevent them from physical shock. In addition, fat has other functions in the body. Some types are used to form a structural component of all body cells. Furthermore, certain vital body

FIGURE 12

CARBOHYDRATE CONTENT OF SOME TYPICAL FOODS

% Carbohydrate

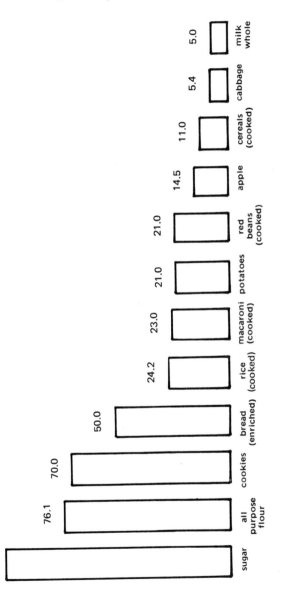

FIGURE 13
METABOLIC FUNCTIONS OF FATS

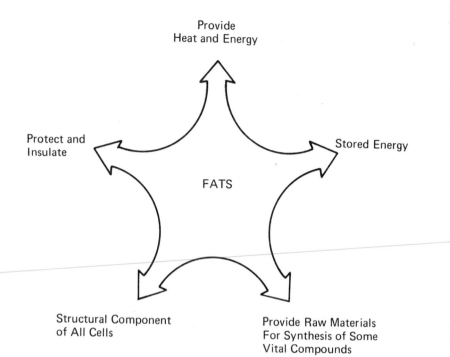

compounds — such as some hormones — are composed of fat-like substances (see Figure 13).

Both plant and animal food contain fat, but the type differs. The fatty acids of animal fats are generally saturated while those of most plant fats are unsaturated, that is, there is room in the fatty acid molecule for other atoms to be added. If there is space for only one pair of atoms it is monounsaturated, but if several pair can be added it is polyunsaturated (see Figure 14). Certain polyunsaturated fatty acids *cannot* be formed within the body from other components and they are considered a dietary essential. Vegetable oils are a rich source of this nutrient. Figure 15 illustrates the percentages of the three types of fatty acids in some typical foods.

The average American diet is considered high in fat and it provides approximately 40 to 45 percent of the dietary energy.[29] The level of fats in the diet appears to increase with increasing affluence, and the biblical description of the wealthy living "off the fat of the land" is as applicable today as it was then. However it is suspected that this fat-rich diet is contributing to the alarming increase in recent years in the incidence of atherosclerosis and the resulting coronary heart disease. Atherosclerosis is characterized by the infiltration of fatty plaques or atheromas into the linings of the arteries, thus restricting blood supply to the heart or other organs. Much research has been devoted to the relationship of diet to this condition, and it is generally believed that a diet rich in animal fats and the fat-like substance cholesterol found with them contributes to the

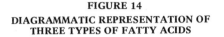

FIGURE 14
DIAGRAMMATIC REPRESENTATION OF
THREE TYPES OF FATTY ACIDS

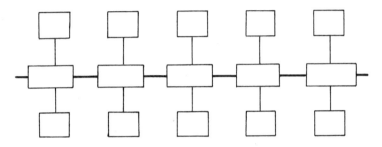

Saturated Fatty Acid

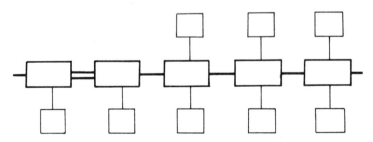

Monounsaturated Fatty Acid

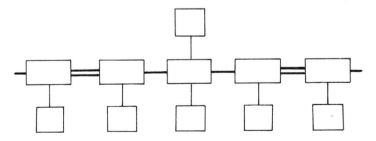

Polyunsaturated Fatty Acid

FIGURE 15

PERCENT OF SATURATED MONOUNSATURATED AND POLYUNSATURATED FATTY ACIDS IN SOME TYPICAL FOODS

% Fatty Acids

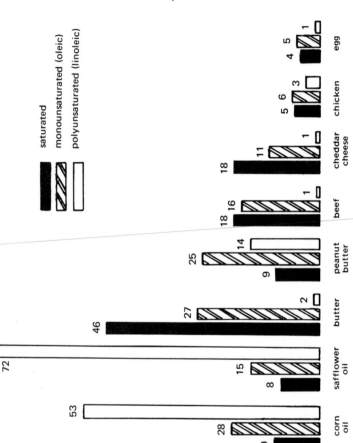

condition.[30] It cannot be said that a high-fat diet alone will cause atherosclerosis as it is believed to be influenced by a combination of factors, however the evidence on the importance of the dietary factor is sufficient enough for the American Heart Association to make the following recommendations to the general public regarding fat intake.

1. To eat less animal (saturated) fat;

2. To increase the intake of unsaturated vegetable oils and other polyunsaturated fats, substituting them for saturated fats wherever possible;

FIGURE 16
TOTAL FAT CONTENT OF SOME TYPICAL FOODS

% Fat

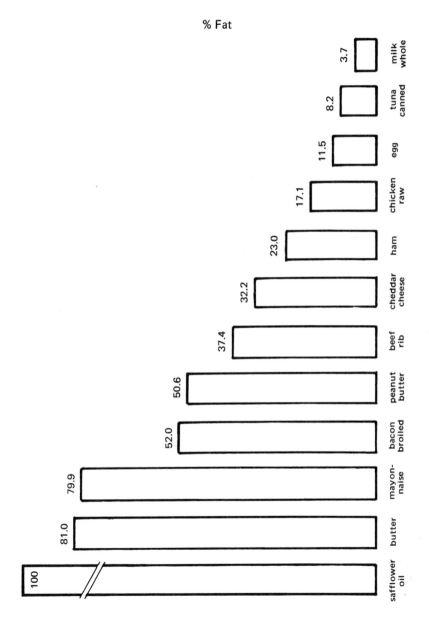

3. To eat less food rich in cholesterol;

4. If overweight, to reduce caloric intake so that desirable weight is achieved and maintained;

5. To apply these dietary recommendations early in life.[31]

Sedentary Americans might well consider reducing their fat intake for two reasons. Fats are a concentrated source of calories and high-fat diets can lead to obesity. Moreover, a high-fat diet may influence the risk of cardiovascular disease. Figure 16 shows the total fat content of some commonly eaten foods.

Minerals. There are fifteen minerals presently known to be needed by the human body. These minerals comprise less than five percent of the total body weight, however they have numerous functions and play an intricate role in metabolic processes. The structural function is their most recognized, for calcium, phosphorus, and small amounts of other minerals are incorporated into bone and tooth cells. Minerals are also essential

FIGURE 17
METABOLIC FUNCTIONS OF MINERALS

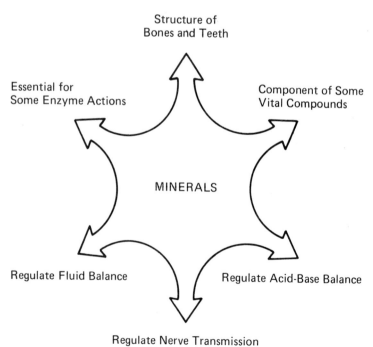

Structure of
Bones and Teeth

Essential for
Some Enzyme Actions

Component of Some
Vital Compounds

MINERALS

Regulate Fluid Balance

Regulate Acid-Base Balance

Regulate Nerve Transmission
And Muscle Contraction

components of vital body compounds, such as iron in hemoglobin and iodine in the hormone thyroxine. In addition, many enzymes either have mineral elements such as copper, zinc, and molybdenum incorporated into their molecular structures or require the presence of certain minerals such as magnesium and manganese to successfully complete chemical reactions. Other functions such as the transmission of nerve impulses, the control of muscle contraction, and the maintenance of body neutrality and normal fluid levels are also influenced by the presence of minerals (see Figure 17). The metabolic functions of minerals are often interrelated, as are the absorption and excretion of different minerals. These interactions are as yet not well-understood, but it seems that often a dietary balance as well as a sufficient supply is essential.[32]

Certain environmental and geographic conditions may result in mineral deficiencies. Simple goiter, which is primarily caused by a deficiency of iodine, is a classic example. In the United States, the Great Lakes region and the Pacific Northwest are goitrous areas because iodine is lacking in the soil. The addition of iodine to table salt caused a rapid decline of the disease, however the incidence has increased somewhat in recent years and is believed to be due to the lack of continuing public education about the benefits of iodized salt. [33]

The Recommended Dietary Allowances gives requirements for five minerals — calcium, phosphorus, iodine, iron, and magnesium (see Appendix B). It is believed that if the diet supplies adequate amounts of the five minerals listed in the RDA, then other mineral requirements will be satisfied. Table 3 shows the rich sources of a number of minerals.

TABLE 3

RICH SOURCES OF SOME MINERALS

Minerals	Rich sources per average serving portion
Calcium	milk, cheese, ice cream, green leafy vegetables*
Phosphorus	liver, milk, meat, cheese, cereals, eggs
Iodine	seafoods, vegetables (grown in soil with iodine), iodized salt
Iron	liver, meat, dried fruits, green leafy vegetables
Magnesium	green leafy vegetables, nuts, whole grain cereals, dried peas and beans

*Excluding spinach, beet greens, and chard.

Vitamins. Vitamins were the last group of nutrients to be discovered, and it is only with the development of microbiology that the cellular functions of vitamins were elucidated. Most vitamins are the major components of coenzymes, the small chemical compounds which assist many enzymes. If the diet is deficient in a vitamin, the needed coenzyme cannot be synthesized, the biochemical reaction it catalyses ceases, and metabolic products pile up at this barrier. These accumulations disrupt body processes and, if severe, result in diseases and eventually death. Some vitamins also appear to act as anti-oxidants and protect unstable nutrients and cellular components from destruction (see Figure 18).

FIGURE 18
METABOLIC FUNCTIONS OF VITAMINS

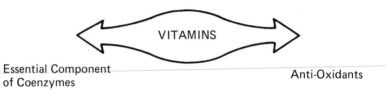

Essential Component of Coenzymes

Anti-Oxidants

Throughout history man has been plagued periodically by vitamin deficiency diseases, for whenever a selection of fruits and vegetables is limited and diets lack variety, these diseases exist (see Table 4). By the 1930's chemists were able to synthesize many vitamins. These could dramatically cure deficiency diseases, and a great deal of enthusiasm was aroused for their use with a wide variety of diseases. Dramatic cures did not result in all the diseases treated, however, and vitamins fell into disrepute. Recently it has been noted that people in even the most affluent societies may be receiving suboptimal amounts, but the effects of this are

TABLE 4
TRADITIONAL VITAMIN DEFICIENCY DISEASES
AND THE MAIN NUTRIENT INVOLVED

Disease	Nutrient
Scurvy	Vitamin C (ascorbic acid)
Beriberi	Vitamin B_1 (thiamine)
Pellagra	Niacin
Rickets	Vitamin D (and calcium)
Xerophthalmia	Vitamin A

not clear. [34] Vitamins, particularly the water soluble ones, are the most labile of all nutrients. The fact that improper storage or preparation of food may destroy their vitamin content further increases the risk of deficiencies when good sources are scarce.

The Recommended Dietary Allowances lists amounts for seven of the water soluble vitamins and three of the fat soluble ones (see Appendix B). Table 5 gives the rich sources of many vitamins.

Water. Water, although seldom thought of as a nutrient, is certainly an essential need. Ten days is probably the survival limit for most individuals without water, whereas men have existed for weeks without food. [35] Water

TABLE 5
RICH SOURCES OF MANY VITAMINS

Vitamins	Rich sources per average serving portion
Water Soluble Vitamins:	
Ascorbic acid (vitamin C)	citrus fruits, cantaloupe, strawberries, broccoli, green leafy vegetables, tomatoes
B vitamins	
Thiamine (B_1)	dried peas and beans, meats (especially pork), cereals (whole grain or enriched), nuts
Riboflavin (B_2)	liver, milk, cheese, eggs, green leafy vegetables
Niacin	liver, meats, dried peas and beans, cereals (whole grain or enriched)
Pyridoxine (B_6)	liver, meats, wheat germ, whole grain cereals
Folic acid	liver, yeast, green leafy vegetables, dried peas and beans, nuts, whole grain cereals
Cobalamin (B_{12})	liver and other organ meats, meats, eggs, milk and milk products
Fat Soluble Vitamins:	
Vitamin A	liver, butter, eggs, whole milk, green and yellow vegetables
Vitamin D	fish liver oils, milk fortified with vitamin D, sunlight
Vitamin E	wheat germ, whole grains, vegetable oils, eggs, whole milk, liver
Vitamin K	green leafy vegetables, egg yolk, soybean oil, liver

has remarkable chemical and physical properties and fulfills a variety of roles in the human body. Most of the nutrients needed by man are soluble in water, and it is a watery fluid that carries these to all cells of the body. In addition, water is an essential internal component of every cell as metabolic reactions take place in the fluids contained within each cell and several biochemical processes require the active chemical participation of water. A variety of physiological mechanisms exist to maintain a balance between these extracellular and intracellular fluids.

Summary. Although each nutrient plays its own role in the body, none acts independently. Cellular metabolism takes place through a series of rapid chemical reactions involving many nutrients at once. A depletion or an overabundance of any one will bring changes in the utilization and metabolism of others, and thus a balance of nutrients is required for optimum functioning. Such a balance can be obtained by eating a variety of foods, and a discussion of the basic types will occupy the remainder of this chapter.

FOODS

Food has always been a major concern of man although its nutritional qualities have not been the most influential factor in his selection of a diet. Man appears to choose food from what is available; he eats what he likes and what seems to agree with him. Early man probably chose from an enormous variety of plant and animal foods ranging from roots and leaves, through grubs and insects, to any larger animals his ingenuity allowed him to capture. Cultural beliefs slowly developed, and in all societies taboos and practices evolved regarding the types of food eaten, methods of production, storage, and preparation as well as restrictions on how and when the food was actually consumed. The food habits which have evolved differ markedly from one culture to another, and what is considered a delicacy in one is often considered unfit for consumption in another. For example, a dietary mainstay of the Masai warriors of Africa is a concoction of cattle blood and milk. Such a fare is repulsive to the average American, yet the consumption of a rare juicy steak enjoyed by individuals in this society is repugnant to the vegetarian Hindu.

Existence is possible on many different types of diet, as nutrients are widely distributed in a variety of edible foods. An optimum diet, however, appears to be much a matter of chance and different cultures have existed at varying levels of health, partially because of their diets. Foods can be naturally divided, according to their nutrient content, into four broad groups: cereals, meats and meat products, milk and dairy products, and

FIGURE 19
A DAILY FOOD GUIDE

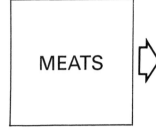

Two or more servings daily

Count as a serving 3 ounces of lean cooked meat, fish, or poultry.

Use eggs, cheese, dry beans, peas, and nuts as alternates.

Four or more servings daily

Count as a serving 1 slice of bread, ½ cup cooked cereal or pasta, and ¾ cup ready-to-eat cereal.

Use whole grain or enriched products.

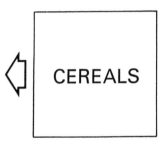

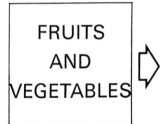

Four or more servings daily

Choose citrus fruits, tomatoes, strawberries, or other vitamin-C-rich fruit daily.

Use dark green or yellow vegetables frequently.

Two or more glasses daily for adults

Three or more glasses daily for children

Four or more glasses daily for teen-agers

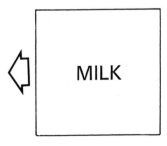

fruits and vegetables. Each group is a good source of certain classes of nutrients but generally lacking in others. Furthermore, within each of these four main groups certain foods may be particularly rich in one or more specific nutrients while others contain lesser amounts. For example, although meat is a good source of proteins and many vitamins and minerals, it is pork that is rich in thiamine, liver that is high in iron, and seafoods that contain iodine. In general, when several different types of food are plentiful, diets are adequate; but when choices are limited, malnutrition may result. Food scientists in the United States have formulated a guide for a balanced diet, giving recommended servings per day for each food group (see Figure 19). Nutritionists of other countries have developed plans suitable to their particular cultural food habits; in general, these are also based on a selection of cereals, meats and animal products as well as fruits and vegetables.

Diversity, it is felt, results in optimal nutrition. Individuals should choose a variety of foods from within each group rather than limiting selections to two or three favorites. Consider, for example, the following possibilities: (1) the selection of cereals such as rice, oats, barley, millet, and corn, as well as wheat and wheat flours; (2) the use of organ meats as well as muscle meats, and the selection of eggs, poultry, fish, and other seafoods; (3) the use of cheeses, yogurt, and other milk products as well as milk; and (4) the selection of a wide variety of vegetables including the leaves, stems, flowers, and roots as well as seeds such as dried peas and beans and nuts, and the choice of a variety of fruits including berries, tree fruits, citrus fruits, and melons. In summary, individuals should choose foods from each of the four broad food groups and diversify within the groups, thus resulting in a balanced diet supplying all essential nutrients.

Cereals. Cereals are a dependable source of calories and are more economical to produce and harvest than animal foods. Cultivation of cereals has probably been the single most important achievement of man, for civilizations developed when he put aside hunting weapons and took up the hoe and a settled way of life. Today, cereals remain the most plentiful source of calories for most cultures. Fortunately they provide vitamins from the B group, minerals such as calcium and iron, and small amounts of proteins as well as energy. Although the protein quality is not as good as that of animal products, when supplemented with small amounts of animal foods both the protein and the flavor of the cereal is enriched. Traditional dishes such as macaroni and cheese, porridge and milk, and spaghetti and meat balls combine cereal and animal foods to supply good-quality protein.

Cereals are often refined. When milling flour the coarse outer layers, rich in protein and B vitamins, as well as the germ are removed, leaving the large inner portion of the seed which consists mostly of starch. Refined products, because of their decreased nutritional qualities, are less susceptible to spoilage by rodents and other pests. However man also loses the benefits of these nutrients, and therefore refined flour is often enriched with iron and several B vitamins, thus partially replacing the nutrients lost during milling. It is important to realize, though, that other cereal products, such as crackers, pasta, cakes, and pastries, are not always made with enriched flours.

The merits of the whole-grain product versus the refined have been debated since the time of classical Greece and Rome, and this debate continues today. It has been shown that when diets consist almost exclusively of unenriched refined grains, deficiency diseases can result, [36] however when the diet is more balanced — as in most industrial societies — it cannot yet be determined whether refined cereals have any adverse effect on health. [37]

The consumption of cereal products in the United States has decreased by 50 to 60 percent in the last century (see Figure 11). In general this has been replaced with sugar, as sugar consumption has more than doubled in that time. With the current concern on reducing weight, bread has been singled out as one of the major contributors to excessive calorie intake. However, one slice of bread supplies only 65 calories. Furthermore, breads and cereals are low in both sugar and fat, another advantage in their favor.

Meats. Man appears to have a natural appetite for meat, and when he can afford it he generally chooses to add more meat to his diet. Americans are no exception, and despite the rising cost of meat, consumption is increasing. Beef is a particular favorite and in 1970 averaged 113 pounds per person, up 2½ pounds from 1969; pork, another favorite, averaged 65.4 pounds per person. [38] Lesser amounts of veal, chicken, and seafoods are consumed.

The proteins of meats and meat products such as eggs are similar to human protein in amino acid composition and liberally supply all the essential amino acids. In addition, meats supply B vitamins, iron, and phosphorus. Different meats vary in their concentrations of specific nutrients and it is recommended that a variety of meats be included in the diet. It is frequently suggested that liver and other organ meats be included once a week specifically for their iron content. The 1965 Food Consumption Survey mentioned above indicated that many diets, particularly those of women and children, were not supplying the recommended daily allowance for iron [39] (see Figure 20).

The fat content of meat varies greatly. Beef, pork, and lamb supply considerable amounts of saturated fats, whereas fish, chicken, veal, and

FIGURE 20

IRON FROM ONE DAY'S DIET
AS A PERCENT OF THE RECOMMENDED ALLOWANCES*

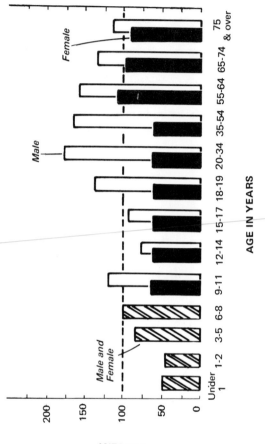

*NAS- NRC, 1968
U.S. Diets of Men, Women, and Children, 1 day in Spring, 1965

From U. S. Department of Agriculture, Agricultural Research Service, Consumer and Food Economics Research Division, *Food intake and nutritive value of diets of men, women, and children in the United States, Spring 1965: A preliminary report.* Washington, D.C.: U.S. Government Printing Office, 1969. P. 7.

128

organ meats have lesser amounts. However, as fat adds flavor and juiciness to meat, in general the fat-rich meats are the most popular. "Prime" beef is marbled with fat and this quality has been encouraged by the cattle industry. Americans would do well to consider increasing their intake of low-fat meats and indulge less in the fat-rich ones.

Milk. Although another meat product, milk is accorded a separate category because of its special nutritional contributions. It provides good-quality protein — although not in the same concentrations as other animal products — carbohydrates in the form of milk sugar, and fat. The B vitamins, particularly riboflavin, the fat-soluble vitamin A, and calcium are also generously supplied. In fact, calcium is one of its major dietary contributions for not only is it one of the few concentrated sources of this nutrient, but the absorption of calcium is assisted by other constituents of milk. The 1965 survey indicated a shortage of calcium, particularly among women (see Figure 21).

In addition to its natural qualities, most milk is fortified by the addition of vitamin D — a nutrient found in only a very few natural foods. The body has the ability to utilize the sun's rays to convert substances in the skin to vitamin D, but in areas of little sunshine or in environments where the sun's rays are blocked by air pollution or crowded housing, a deficiency of vitamin D often results in rickets, a body-deforming disease of children. Fortification of milk with vitamin D has almost eliminated this disease.

Fresh milk is easily contaminated and spoiled, and throughout history man has devised various ways to overcome this, resulting in a variety of cheeses as well as buttermilk, yogurt, and other soured and fermented milks. Although cheese is a milk product, it is a more concentrated source of protein than the fluid milks and thus may also be used as a substitute for meat. Butter, made from milk fat, contains the fat-soluble vitamin A. Margarine, a butter substitute, is of equal nutritive value when fortified with vitamin A. It is made from vegetable oils which have been hardened by adding hydrogen to some of the polyunsaturated fatty acids. Different margarines vary in the degree of this hydrogenation. Many are labeled with the P/S ratio, which is an indication of the proportion of polyunsaturated fats to saturated fats. As a general rule, however, the softer the margarine when chilled, the higher the percentage of unsaturated fats.

When controlling the fat and calorie content of the diet, the use of skimmed milk or partially skimmed milk is recommended. Those skimmed milk products which are fortified with vitamin A should be selected for this vitamin is lost when the milk fat is removed.

FIGURE 21

CALCIUM FROM ONE DAY'S DIET
AS A PERCENT OF THE RECOMMENDED ALLOWANCES*

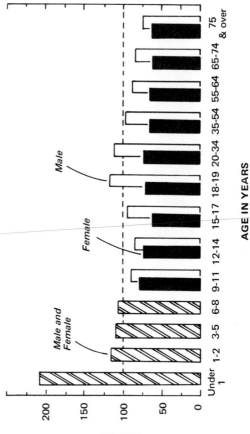

*NAS-NRC, 1968
U.S. Diets of Men, Women, and Children, 1 day in Spring, 1965

From U. S. Department of Agriculture, Agricultural Research Service, Consumer and Food Economics Research Division, *Food intake and nutritive value of diets of men, women, and children in the United States, Spring 1965: A preliminary report.* Washington, D.C.: U.S. Government Printing Office, 1969. P. 6.

Fruits and Vegetables. Fruits and vegetables make valuable nutrient contributions to the diet for they provide certain nutrients not found in the other three groups, especially vitamin C and carotene, a substance the body can convert to vitamin A. This food group also supplies calcium and iron as well as small amounts of other minerals. Most of these foods are low in the energy-yielding nutrients — carbohydrates, fats, and proteins — hence they supply only small amounts of calories.

Both dark green leafy vegetables such as kale, Swiss chard, and spinach as well as such yellow vegetables as carrots and squash are more generously endowed with vitamins and minerals than many other vegetables. The 1965 Food Consumption Survey indicated, however, that only 10 to 20 percent of the people interviewed ate these vegetables during the period of the survey, a decrease since 1955.[40] The use of a variety of vegetables is to be encouraged both for their unique nutrient content and for their low energy value. Attempts perhaps have to be made to make them more appealing and interesting by the use of herbs, spices, flavoring salts, lemon juice, and interesting combinations of both raw and cooked vegetables.

Vegetable seeds such as peas, beans, and lentils contain more protein as well as more carbohydrates than other vegetables and can be used as economical substitutes for meats. They should, however, be combined with small amounts of meat or meat products to enhance their protein quality.

Fruits are more popular than vegetables although most do not supply the same concentration of vitamins and minerals. Their main contribution is vitamin C. This vitamin is easily destroyed by both heat and oxidative processes, but fortunately certain constituents of fruits and the fact that they often are not cooked help to prevent the destruction of this sensitive nutrient. Citrus fruits, strawberries, melons, and tomatoes are all excellent sources of this vitamin. Fruits also contain some minerals, and yellow fruits supply carotene as well. Fruits are recommended for weight loss regimes for they can take the place of rich and often non-nutritious desserts. Raw apple slices sprinkled with cinnamon may not have quite the same appeal as apple pie with ice cream, but the comparison of 40 calories to 500 calories makes them a worthy consideration.

Other Foods. The four basic food groups discussed above all provide the body with nutrients as well as energy. Other foods particularly relished by affluent societies provide energy but lack other nutrients. These foods, called "empty calorie foods," are comprised of sucrose, pure animal fats, and combinations of these with unrefined white flour. In societies where strenuous physical work is necessary and caloric needs are high, tastes for these foods could be indulged. In sedentary populations, however, excessive use of such foods leads to obesity and may contribute to degenerative diseases of the arteries and heart. Furthermore, such food habits frequently crowd out other nutritious foods in the diet.

To resist the temptations of these empty calorie foods is not an easy matter, as they are available everywhere. The snack-type foods such as potato chips, soda pop, and candy are often the most readily available foods outside the home. Indeed, vending machines, snack bars, and entertainment centers generally offer little else, and it has become habit for the consumption of these foods to accompany many leisure-time activities. Americans appear to be consuming snack foods in increasing amounts. The 1965 Food Consumption Survey showed an 83 percent increase in potato chip consumption since the 1955 survey.[41] The use of carbonated beverages and fruit ades and punches is also increasing, and in 1966 the National Soft Drink Association reported that an average American drinks about 18 gallons of these drinks yearly.[42] Furthermore, convenience foods allow instant preparation of such calorie-rich treats as deep fat fried foods, desserts rich in fat and sugar, elaborate pastries, and other baked products.

The consumption of alcoholic beverages can also add many empty calories to the diet, often unknowingly. It has been estimated that in the United States an average of 76 calories per day are provided by alcohol,[43] exclusive of the drinks with which they are mixed. By excluding children, teetotalers, and occasional drinkers, it is evident that alcohol is providing a considerable proportion of calories to the diets of some people. Wine and other alcoholic beverages enhance mealtimes, sociability, and relaxation; nonetheless, it is necessary to recognize their contribution of calories and use them in moderation.

CONCLUSION

In a society where the need for physical exertion is minimal, food energy must be controlled to avoid obesity. A wise selection of foods is essential in order to accomplish this and yet provide liberal amounts of the nutrients needed to contribute to long-term health, defined by the World Health Organization as "a state of complete physical, mental, and social well-being and not merely the absence of stress or infirmity."[44]

A nutritious diet does not mean uninteresting meals and a rigid regime for eating is a pleasure and must remain so. Pleasing foods and creative cooking can still be enjoyed, and the satisfactions of a glass of wine with dinner and the inclusion of a tasty light dessert do not have to be denied. It is recommended, however, that empty calorie foods should be used sparingly and that the majority of foods be chosen from the four major food groups. Variety and creativity can be used to create interesting, nutritious meals and enhance the natural flavors of foods. It is this same plan which forms the basis of a successful weight reduction program.

FOOTNOTES

1. Farber, M., Wilson, N. L., Wilson, R., and Wilson, H. L. *Food and civilization: A symposium.* Springfield, Ill., Charles C. Thomas, 1962.
2. Burgess, A. and Dean, R. F. A. *Malnutrition and food habits.* London: Tavistock, 1962.
3. *White House Conference on Food, Nutrition, and Health: Final report.* Washington, D.C.: U. S. Government Printing Office, 1970. P. 51.
4. U. S. Department of Agriculture, Agricultural Research Service, Consumer and Food Economics Research Division. *Food intake and nutritive value of diets of men, women, and children in the United States, Spring 1965: A preliminary report.* Washington, D.C.: U. S. Government Printing Office, 1969.
5. Adelson, S. F. Changes in diets of households, 1955 to 1965. *Journal of Home Economics,* 1968, *60,* 448-455.
6. Schaefer, A. E. Prepared statement. In *Nutrition and human needs—1970: Hearings before the Select Committee on Nutrition and Human Needs of the United States Senate.* Part 3. Washington, D.C.: U. S. Government Printing Office, 1970.
7. Guthrie, H. A. *Introductory nutrition. St. Louis, Mo.: C. V. Mosby, 1967.*
8. Kannel, W. B. The disease of living. *Nutrition Today,* 1971, *6*(3), 2-11.
9. *Ibid.*
10. The American way of death. *Scientific American,* 1971, *224*(5), 44.
11. Kannel, *op. cit.*
12. Lewis, I. J. Government investment in health care. *Scientific American,* 1971, *224*(4), 17-25.
13. Shank, R. E. A chink in our armour. *Nutrition Today,* 1970, *5*(2), 2-11.
14. National Research Council, Food and Nutrition Board, Committee on Maternal Nutrition. *Maternal nutrition and the course of pregnancy: Summary report.* Washington, D.C.: National Academy of Sciences, 1970. P. 15.
15. Scrimshaw, N. S., Taylor, C. E., and Gordon, J. E. *Interactions of nutrition and infection.* Geneva: World Health Organization, 1968.
16. Kruse, H. D. *Nutrition, its meaning, scope and significance.* Springfield, Ill.: Charles C. Thomas, 1969.
17. Watson, James D. *Molecular biology of the gene.* New York: W. A. Benjamin, 1965.
18. Davidson, S. and Passmore, R. *Human nutrition and dietetics.* Edinburgh: E. and S. Livingstone, 1969.
19. U. S. Department of Agriculture, *op. cit.*
20. Brown, D. W. Present knowledge of protein nutrition. In *Present knowledge in nutrition.* New York: The Nutrition Foundation, 1967.
21. Briggs, G. M. Letter to the editor. *Nutrition Reviews,* 1965, *23,* 95.
22. Bloom, W. L. and Azar, G. J. Similarities of carbohydrate deficiency and fasting. *Archives of Internal Medicine,* 1963, *112,* 333-343.
23. Hodges, R. E. Present knowledge of carbohydrates. In *Present knowledge in nutrition, op. cit.*
24. Duncan, G. G. (Ed.) *Diseases of metabolism.* Philadelphia: W. B. Saunders, 1964.
25. Shaw, J. H. Present knowledge of nutrition and dental caries. In *Present knowledge in nutrition, op. cit.*
26. MacDonald, I. Physiological role of dietary carbohydrate. *World Review of Nutrition and Dietetics,* 1967, *8,* 143-183.
27. Yudkin, J. Sucrose and heart disease. *Nutrition Today,* 1969, *4*(1), 16-20.
28. U. S. Department of Agriculture, Economic Research Service. U. S. food consumption: Sources of data and trends. In *Statistical Bulletin, No. 364.* Washington, D.C.: U. S. Government Printing Office, 1965.
29. *Ibid.*
30. International cooperative study on cardiovascular epidemiology. *Nutrition Reviews,* 1970, *28,* 281-285.
31. Blakeslee, A. and Stamler, J. *Your heart has nine lives.* New York: Pocket Books, 1966. P. vii.
32. Essential inorganic elements in nutrition: Functions and inter-relationships. *Dairy Council Digest,* 1968, *39,* 5.

33. Iodized salt: A staff report. *Nutrition Today,* 1969, 4(1), 22-25.
34. Marks, J. *Vitamins in health and disease: A modern reappraisal.* London: Churchill, 1968.
35. Davidson and Passmore, *op. cit.*
36. Bogert, J. L., Briggs, G. M., and Calloway, D. H. *Nutrition and physical fitness.* Philadelphia: W. B. Saunders, 1966.
37. Davidson and Passmore, *op. cit.*
38. Associated Press release, 1970.
39. U. S. Department of Agriculture, *Food intake, op. cit.*
40. *Ibid.*
41. U. S. Department of Agriculture. *Food for us all: Yearbook of agriculture.* Washington, D.C.: U. S. Government Printing Office, 1969.
42. *Ibid.*
43. Farber *et al.,op. cit.*
44. Pike, M. *Food and society.* New York: International Publications Service, 1968. P. 33.

NUTRITION MANAGEMENT PROGRAM

O, that this too too solid flesh would melt,
Thaw and resolve itself into a dew! [1]

This fervent desire of Hamlet is undoubtedly shared by the 40 million or so Americans currently fighting the "battle of the bulge," much time, energy, and enthusiasm have been devoted to the search for a diet that will lead to an easy and rapid loss of excess body fat. Low-carbohydrate diets, high-fat diets, and both low- and high-protein diets have all been hailed at various times as the answer to the weight-control problem. However, to date there is no evidence to recommend any of these over a diet balanced in carbohydrates, fats, and protein.

The origin of low-carbohydrate diets can be traced to the 1800's, and they appear to maintain an eternal appeal for those attempting weight reduction.[2] They have been given a variety of names—the Mayo diet, the Du Pont diet and, with the addition of alcohol, the "drinking man's" diet. Such diets inevitably result in either a high-fat or a combined high fat/high protein regimen. Some low-carbohydrate diets have been claimed to lead to weight loss even with unlimited calories, however investigators have demonstrated that such diets must be deficient in calories if body fat stores are to be used.[3] Although the first ten days on a low-carbohydrate regimen may result in a rapid loss of body weight, investigations[4] conducted under controlled conditions in metabolic units have indicated that this loss is due to reduction of body fluids as well as body fat. In addition, they have shown that when the regimen is continued, the rate of weight loss decreases, and after three weeks weight loss is no greater than on isocaloric diets either high in carbohydrate content or balanced in carbohydrates, fats, and protein. The survey results of approximately 1,500 British physicians support these metabolic laboratory findings. The doctors reported that diets restricting carbohydrates resulted in no greater effectiveness than diets restricting fats in the treatment of their obese patients.[5] When this is considered in light of the finding that carbohydrates are probably a necessary component of the diet, the absence of which can result in fluid and electrolyte imbalances, ketosis, and fatigue,[6] it should be clear that diets overly restricted in this nutrient should be avoided. While the Food and Nutrition Board of the National Research Council does not list a specific Recommended Dietary Allowance for carbohydrates, they do recommend that diets include at least 100 grams (400 carbohydrate calories) of this nutrient daily.[7]

A second type of diet, the low-protein diet, has also been popular at times. This often involves the replacement of protein in the diet with an increase in carbohydrate foods. The banana and skim milk diet and the rice diet are two extreme examples. Another low-protein diet, called "the Rockefeller diet," was developed originally for experimental purposes in hospital metabolic units and was not intended for the wide general-public use that resulted—a fate common to other experimental dietary regimens as well.

A diet moderately high in protein content is frequently recommended for weight-reduction regimens. The majority of adult diets provide between 10 and 15 percent of their daily calories in the form of protein,[8] however, more liberal amounts are commonly believed to increase dietary satiety as digestion, absorption, and utilization of proteins proceeds at a comparatively slow rate. The diets described and supplied with this management program provide approximately 20 percent of their total calories in the form of protein, thus taking advantage of possible increased satiety values. As a precautionary measure, however, dieters are advised to increase their consumption of those protein foods that are reasonably low in fat content as protein-rich diets may result in inadvertent increases in dietary saturated fat content as well.

A very high protein diet is currently popular in which the protein content greatly exceeds commonly consumed amounts. The basis of such diets is generally the belief that they "burn up" more calories or increase metabolism to a greater extent than other diets. The utilization of food within the body does result in an increase in metabolism over basal needs, called the Specific Dynamic Action (SDA) of foods, an effect which has been compared to the increased glow of a fire when fuel is added. Normal mixed diets containing carbohydrates, fats, and protein result in an approximate increase in metabolism of 6 percent.[9] When proteins *alone* are consumed a considerable increase in metabolism results, however a purely protein diet is not feasible under normal circumstances; indeed, it is difficult to radically increase the dietary protein content as they are not found in the same concentrations in foods as are carbohydrates and fats. SDA has proven to be relatively constant despite moderately wide variations in dietary protein.[10] Animal experiments indicate that *both* an *insufficiency* and an *overabundance* of protein may increase the SDA,[11] however such manipulation in the human diet may result in imbalances and inadequacies of other dietary nutrients. In general, the SDA of food is perhaps overemphasized[12] with respect to its metabolic benefits to dieters, as such effects are insignificant when compared to the increases caused by even minimal muscular exertion. For example, merely changing from a lying to a sitting position may increase metabolism approximately 20 percent[13] and thus has a far greater effect on energy expenditure than the SDA of food. It is suggested, therefore, that dieters might find it more profitable to increase their total metabolism through increased physical exertion rather than through radical manipulations of the protein content of their diet.

Each of the above diets has its proponents and underlying theory, and in addition many have unique limitations. In general, those that attempt to radically alter proportions of the three main dietary components—carbohydrates, fats, and protein—suffer two major drawbacks. First, while radical changes may have a temporary psychological appeal, experience has shown that extreme alterations in existing food practices cannot be tolerated for long periods of time. Such diets therefore are not conducive to the long-term regimens necessary for the reconditioning of eating habits and maintenance of weight reduction. Second, bizarre regimens may fail to provide satisfactory levels of essential nutrients.

Ideally a dietary management program should provide a reasonable balance of carbohydrates, fats, and protein, should restrict calories moderately but provide a generous supply of all other essential nutrients, and in addition should consider cultural and individual food preferences. The remainder of this chapter will describe a means of incorporating these considerations into individualized dietary plans. To facilitate adherence to these plans, techniques will also be described for the monitoring of food intake and for the preparation of foods to result in minimum caloric content yet maximum palatability.

DIETARY MANAGEMENT PLAN

The dietary management plan advanced here makes it possible to (a) control the caloric content of the daily diet, (b) ensure a nutritious diet, (c) allow for individual preferences and customs, and (d) permit individual participation in menu planning. The plan is based upon a division of the main food groups into lists, each list containing a variety of foods approximately equal in food value (see Appendix C). Dieters are allowed a selection of foods from each list, the type and number being in accordance with sound nutritional levels and determined by the caloric limitations of the chosen food plan. Foods in a list are called exchanges as they may be freely exchanged for other foods in the same list.

Systems of food exchanges have proven successful for many health problems requiring dietary changes, such as diets for diabetics and cardiovascular patients, and they have formed the basis for successful long-term weight-reduction regimens.[14] Their success may be attributed to three factors. First, they allow for individual likes and dislikes, thus all dieters are not restricted to the same "1/2 grapefruit, boiled egg" breakfast menu common to many diets. Secondly, they permit individual participation in the decision-making processes of food selection and meal planning, factors which research has demonstrated result in increased satisfaction and stronger commitment to changes in food habits.[15] Finally, they allow a retention of appropriate eating practices yet provide the opportunity for needed change, and experience has shown that successful dietary changes are best achieved by blending needed changes with existing practices.[16] Thus, within the food exchange framework the Italian may retain his pasta, the Oriental his rice, and the American his bread, each according to his own customs and preferences.

The calorie decision. The first step in weight reduction is the establishment of a caloric deficit which will result in a satisfactory, continuous weight loss. As a general rule, it is recommended that weight-reducers adopt a target of approximately one to two pounds per week. There are several reasons for this. First, it has been shown that successful dieters tend to lose between 1.4 and .69 pounds per week, the smaller rate of weight loss tending to be found at later stages of the reducing program.[17] Second, it has been estimated that weight loss requiring diets involving less than 1,200 calories may be maladapted to the social pressures commonly found to operate upon eating[18] as well as to the physiological stresses of hunger; in addition, they may fail to provide an adequately balanced nutritional intake. Severely restricted diets may also result in a physiological accommodation to the reduced food intake by a reduction in energy expenditure.[19] Finally, rapid weight loss would appear to conflict with the gradual process of weight accretion and perhaps contribute to a disturbance in a homeostatic balance at some level; it is often followed by rapid weight gain seemingly as a compensatory reaction.[20] For these reasons it is recommended that dieters limit their weight loss to one pound weekly through restriction of caloric intake, additional weight loss being achieved through increases in energy output. (An exercise management plan is provided in Chapter 7.)

One pound of body fat can be lost by creating a caloric deficit of 3,500 calories; thus a daily reduction of 500 calories would result in a weekly loss of 1 pound (7 days x 500 calories per day), providing of course that energy expenditure remains constant. To calculate the amount of daily caloric intake necessary for such a weight loss, two steps should be followed. First, reference to Table 1 will determine the estimated daily caloric requirement for individuals of given ages and sex, assuming that energy expenditure needs can be classified as light—involving neither wholly sedentary nor vigorously active lives. Second, 500 calories should be subtracted from the value obtained by reference to the table. The needs of each individual may vary somewhat from these figures as the caloric requirements listed in Table 1 are for persons of average height and weight. Nevertheless the caloric level calculated from the table provides a reasonable approximation of the number of calories needed for weight loss. The ideal test of this estimate, however, is trial and dieters should carefully monitor their personal experience with weight loss and caloric restriction as illustrated in Chapter 3 (Figure 5), adjusting caloric intake as needed. Furthermore, as each 25 pounds is lost, it is necessary to *decrease* caloric intake by an additional 100 calories because less energy is required to move around a lighter body mass.[21]

TABLE 1

CALORIC ALLOWANCE
FOR DIFFERENT AGE GROUPS

	Age 22-35	Age 35-55	Age 55-75 +
Males	2,800	2,600	2,400
Females	2,000	1,850	1,700

Adapted from National Research Council, Food and Nutrition Board, *Recommended Dietary Allowances.* (Publication 1694, 7th rev. ed.) Washington, D.C.: National Academy of Sciences, 1968. P. 102.

Food exchanges. Foods have been divided into five lists: meats, cereals, milk, vegetables, and fruits (see Appendix C). Each of the foods within a list, in the amount recommended, is similar in nutrient content and caloric value to all other foods in the *same* list. For example, both one slice of bread and 1/2 cup of cooked rice are on the cereal exchange list. Each of these supplies approximately 70 calories of energy, and they contain similar amounts of carbohydrates, proteins, vitamins, and minerals. Either may be chosen for one cereal exchange.

In addition to the five exchange lists based on food groups, there is a sixth food exchange list—the miscellaneous foods. These include concentrated sources of fats and sugars, as well as alcoholic beverages, which are commonly eaten and enjoyed in modern societies. The pitfalls of overindulgence in such foods have been discussed, but because they are an established part of the existing cultural food patterns, it is improbable that such foods can be totally excluded. Indeed, food plans attempting to do this may, in the long run, be doomed to failure.

It must be pointed out that the nutrient and caloric values of the foods within a food exchange list are not identical; to a degree, exactness is sacrificed for simplicity and convenience. Caloric values, however, are always approximations. Steaks of the same weight but from different animals will vary in caloric content, as will measures of wheat grown in different soils. Spaghetti prepared by different cooks will not have the same caloric value. For absolutely accurate calculations, laboratory analysis of each individual food eaten is needed, but for practical purposes, calculations based on food-exchange caloric values are sufficiently accurate, quickly done, and used by most professionals for approximating daily caloric intake.[22]

Until portions of food can be estimated accurately, it is essential to measure or weigh the food before eating. Most foods on the exchange lists can be measured with regular kitchen measuring spoons, measuring cups, or a ruler (see Appendix D for a list of equivalents). Many meat exchanges, however, are listed by weight, and an inexpensive postal scale is accurate and easy to use. Most meat exchanges weigh 1 ounce; however, an average serving portion of meat for dinner weighs 3 or 4 ounces, thus equaling 3 or 4 meat exchanges. The weights of the exchanges are for cooked meat, with 4 ounces of raw meat weighing approximately 3 ounces when cooked.

In summary, then, the six food exchange lists are as follows:

1. Meat exchange list
2. Cereal exchange list
3. Milk exchange list
4. Vegetable exchange list
5. Fruit exchange list
6. Miscellaneous exchange list

In addition, several beverages and food items, such as tea, coffee, clear soups, herbs, seasonings, and certain raw vegetables supply negligible amounts of calories to the diet. These can be eaten in unlimited quantities. The complete food exchange lists can be found in Appendix C; abbreviated lists are also available with the book and should be placed in the vinyl folder.

Special diet foods. It will be noted that specific suggestions have not been made for the inclusion of special "diet" foods. There are three reasons why this has not been done. First, the goal of this regimen is to recondition eating habits rather than to substitute low-calorie foods or chemicals for those foods or nutrients, such as sugars and fats, that have contributed to the obese state. Second, the long-term effects on body health and function resulting from frequent use of many of these substitutes is not known. The sugar substitute cyclamate was removed from the market once animal experiments suggested it could be potentially harmful to man. Finally, some of the special diet foods still contain considerable energy value and are misleading. For example, many of the "diet breads" are merely sliced more thinly than the regular bread and other diet foods reduce only salt content and not calories, which may have some effect on body water content but does not aid in reducing body fat stores.

Undoubtedly some special "diet" foods will help make the process of dieting and changing eating habits easier. It is recommended, however, that the calorie content listed on the label of these foods be checked, and that, like other foods, they be measured accurately. It may be necessary to record such foods as an exchange or part of an exchange on the daily food plan, or they may have to be added as an extra food. Moreover, it is suggested that the savings in calories be compared with the increased cost of many of these foods.

Food plans. The second step of the dietary management plan is the choice of a food plan, based on food exchanges, which will be close in caloric value to the previously calculated amount needed to result in a weekly one pound loss of weight. The following diets range from 1,200 to 2,300 calories per day. Each provides approximately 20 percent of its calories as protein and averages 30 percent of its calories as fats—a proportion in line with current theories regarding dietary fat content; the remainder is obtained in carbohydrates, preferably in the form of starch rather than sucrose. These diets are accurate to within 20 calories of the amounts specified.

1,200 calorie daily food plan

6 meat exchanges
4 cereal exchanges
2 milk exchanges
3 vegetable exchanges
3 fruit exchanges
3 exchanges from miscellaneous list

1,350 calorie daily food plan

6 meat exchanges
5 cereal exchanges
2 milk exchanges
3 vegetables exchanges
4 fruit exchanges
4 exchanges from miscellaneous list

1,500 calorie daily food plan

7 meat exchanges
5 cereal exchanges
2 milk exchanges
3 vegetable exchanges
5 fruit exchanges
5 exchanges from miscellaneous list

1,700 calorie daily food plan

8 meat exchanges
6 cereal exchanges
2 milk exchanges
3 vegetable exchanges
5 fruit exchanges
6 exchanges from miscellaneous list

1,900 calorie daily food plan

9 meat exchanges
7 cereal exchanges
2 milk exchanges
3 vegetable exchanges
6 fruit exchanges
7 exchanges from miscellaneous list

2,100 calorie daily food plan

9 meat exchanges
8 cereal exchanges
3 milk exchanges
3 vegetable exchanges
6 fruit exchanges
8 exchanges from miscellaneous list

2,300 calorie daily food plan

10 meat exchanges
9 cereal exchanges
3 milk exchanges
3 vegetable exchanges
6 fruit exchanges
9 exchanges from miscellaneous list

These diets may be modified somewhat to suit individual preferences and budgets. As can be seen in the food exchange lists (Appendix C), each meat exchange provides approximately 75 calories of energy, while each cereal exchange yields approximately 70 calories. Therefore, cereal exchanges to a degree may be substituted for meat exchanges as an economical measure, or meat exchanges used in place of cereal to accommodate personal preferences. Both fruit exchanges and exchanges from the miscellaneous list supply 40 calories. Since some persons may wish to increase or decrease their consumption of fruit, these may be exchanged to a limited extent for miscellaneous foods. Although deviations from the suggested food plans are possible, the following minimum selections should be followed to maintain a balanced diet.

6 meat exchanges
3 cereal exchanges
2 milk exchanges
2 vegetable exchanges
2 fruit exchanges

It is advised that the daily food be divided into at least three meals with allowances made for snacks. The obese person often has a history of eating most of his or her food in the latter part of the day, with a tendency to overeat considerably at this time.[23] When the point of hunger (not just appetite) is reached, uncontrolled and indiscriminate eating often results. Therefore *breakfast is strongly recommended, as eating in the early part of the day appears to help control eating throughout the day.* Furthermore, research with animals suggests that an added advantage to frequent meals may be that some energy is "wasted" when the daily calories are ingested in *frequent* meals rather than when the same number are condensed into one large meal.[24] The food plan charts provided in the vinyl folder distribute the allowed number of food exchanges on each diet into three meals a day, however this is simply a guide to suggest a practical way for the daily food allotments to be distributed. As suggested in Chapter 3 food allotments from each meal can be saved for snacks if this proves to be a successful way of alleviating feelings of hunger or deprivation. In addition, the foods which supply negligible amounts of calories, called calorie-free foods, can also be used for snacks.

MONITORING THE DIET

Eating records. Once an appropriate diet is chosen, the monitoring of food intake is a third step in dietary management. It is essential to record the amount of food eaten in order to provide (a) self-feedback as to how much more can be eaten while remaining within the chosen dietary program; (b) cues for the selection of appropriate foods; and (c) means of obtaining help from others in monitoring what is eaten. Although most conventional nutrition management programs recommend this recording procedure, there are several pitfalls. For instance, if food consumption is recorded at the end of the day, memory may be faulty and the records inaccurate. On the other hand, if it is necessary to write detailed information whenever food is eaten, this tedious task may be neglected. To be optimally useful, therefore, an eating record must be quickly and simply kept and provide immediate, readily available information.

The vinyl folder included with this book gives the dieter a means of readily securing the information essential to effective dietary management. The chosen daily food plan card (found at the back of the book) is inserted, face up, in the folder. As each meal or snack is eaten, the type and number of food exchanges consumed should be indicated on the vinyl folder by writing the time at which a food is eaten in the corresponding rectangular box on the underlying daily food plan (see Figure 1). Be *certain* to use the *transparency marking pen* provided, as records may then be erased daily with a damp kleenex or cloth. This will then permit the reuse of the vinyl envelope indefinitely.

FIGURE 1

DAILY FOOD PLAN WITH
SAMPLE RECORDING OF INTAKE

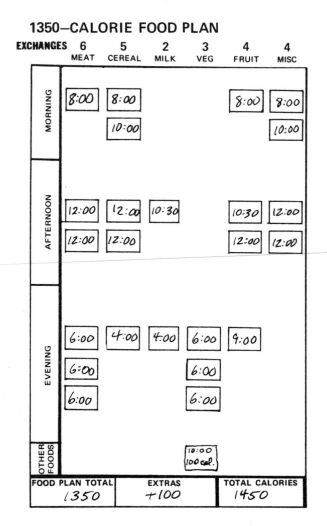

Although the consumption of extra food is not encouraged, it must be recorded on the folder in the space marked OTHER FOODS. Calculate the calorie content of such extras by referring to the exchange food lists (Appendix C) or, if the extra is not included there, check the calorie chart in Appendix E. Add these extra calories to those allowed on the calorie food plan and record the total daily calories in the space for TOTAL CALORIES. For example, a woman on a 1,350-calorie diet might record her daily food as in Figure 1.

Adjustments of the basic food plan can be recorded merely by drawing arrows as shown in Figure 2, bearing in mind that the caloric levels of the foods exchanged should be approximately equal. Here a 1,500-calorie diet has been adjusted to account for a preference for foods from the meat exchange list. The arrows from cereals to meats indicate the substitution of two meat exchanges for two cereal exchanges.

Graphing. As a final management step, it is necessary at the end of the day to record the total calories on the Eating-Weight-Exercise graph described in Chapter 3 (Figure 5) and available with the book. It is recommended that individuals weigh themselves at the same time every day, preferably in the morning, before dressing but after voiding, as weight is at its lowest at this point. Recording this weight on the Eating-Weight-Exercise graph permits a comparison of the fluctuations in the amount of food eaten, energy expended, and weight change.

Since daily weight fluctuations are affected by fluid loss and retention, irregular bowel habits, and irregularities of the scales, the graph will seldom be linear. This is normal. It is entirely possible for fat to be lost but for weight to remain unchanged for several days. (Women, especially, experience fluid retention related to the menstrual cycle.) Although this often leads to discouragement and abandoning of the diet, if the diet is continued, weight loss inevitably follows such plateaus. Figure 3 illustrates a weight-loss pattern on a calorie-controlled diet in the metabolic ward of a hospital. Daily fluctuations exist, however the overall graph of weight loss is linear.

FOOD PREPARATION TIPS

As well as making changes in the types and amounts of foods selected, an adjunct to the management program may be the need for changes in food preparation methods as well. As a general rule, when buying foods the less preparation and processing a food has undergone, the less chance there is of hidden calories being present. For example, canned fruit and fruit juices with added sugar have more calories than the fresh

FIGURE 2

**1500-CALORIE FOOD PLAN SHOWING
ADJUSTMENTS FOR INDIVIDUAL PREFERENCES**

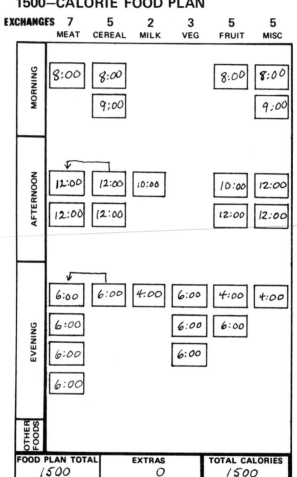

1500—CALORIE FOOD PLAN

EXCHANGES	7	5	2	3	5	5
	MEAT	CEREAL	MILK	VEG	FRUIT	MISC

	MEAT	CEREAL	MILK	VEG	FRUIT	MISC
MORNING	8:00	8:00 / 9:00			8:00	8:00 / 9:00
AFTERNOON	12:00 / 12:00	12:00 / 12:00	10:00		10:00 / 12:00	12:00 / 12:00
EVENING	6:00 / 6:00 / 6:00 / 6:00	6:00	4:00	6:00 / 6:00 / 6:00	4:00 / 6:00	4:00
OTHER FOODS						

FOOD PLAN TOTAL	EXTRAS	TOTAL CALORIES
1500	0	1500

FIGURE 3

**ACTUAL (SOLID LINE) AND PREDICTED (DOTTED LINE)
WEIGHT LOSS FOR 19-YEAR-OLD GIRL,
175.5 CM (5 FT 9 INCHES) TALL**

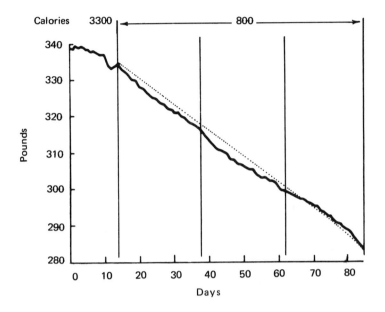

Reproduced with permission from W. M. Bortz, Predictability of weight loss.
Journal of the American Medical Association, 1968, *204*, 102.

product. Sugar-coated cereals have more food energy than uncooked cereals and are more expensive as well. Potato chips are far more caloric than boiled or baked potatoes. In addition, when food bulk is removed during processing there is a tendency to eat *more* of the resulting product. A small baked potato will be satisfying while an equivalent amount of instant mashed potatoes likely will not. And a whole apple appears to be more food and takes more time to eat than the equivalent four ounces of apple juice. Finally, with unprocessed foods more of the original nutrient content remains. With each exposure to heat and other influences during processing, valuable nutrients may be destroyed.

Preparing meals while controlling calorie content does not have to result in less appetizing or less creative meals. Seasonings, herbs, and juices of both fruits and vegetables can be used to enhance the natural flavors of basic foods. The purchase of a low-calorie cookbook will offer many suggestions and ideas for exciting and interesting low-calorie recipes and meals. With time, the appetite becomes trained to appreciate and prefer less rich foods.

The following suggestions briefly outline how foods on the food exchange lists can be prepared so as to keep the calorie level low, but the taste and nutritional quality high.

Meat Exchanges

1. Increase the use of the leaner meats, seafoods, cottage cheese, and skim milk cheeses.

2. Always cut all visible fat from meat before cooking and cook without adding extra fat.

3. Remove the skin from poultry before eating, as a layer of fat lies attached to the skin. White meat has less natural fat than the moister dark meat.

4. Buy water-packed canned fish or rinse oil from fish with hot water before using.

5. Use lemon juice, herbs, or onion flakes with seafood dishes for added flavor and variety. Fish is an economical and low-fat meat exchange.

6. Use seasoned tomato juice or bouillon in meat, fish, and poultry recipes instead of creamed gravies and rich sauces.

7. Try cooking with dry wines. Most of the calorie-rich alcohol evaporates in the cooking but leaves a flavorful sauce. Sweet wines, however, contain more sugar and have more calories.

8. Try combining meat and fruit for flavor variations. Pineapple with chicken or apples with ham are two suggestions.

9. To encourage the use of organ meats, try combining smaller amounts of them with other meats. Liver with ham and steak with kidney are two possibilities.

Cereal Exchanges

1. Try a variety of breads—herb, whole wheat, rye, cheese, cinnamon, and spiced breads— to add interest to meals. A slice of cinnamon toast and fruit can substitute for a rich dessert.

2. Try making homemade bread. It will be appreciated as much or more than home-prepared calorie-rich desserts.

3. Carbohydrate-rich vegetables are included in the cereal exchange list. Dried peas, beans, and lentils when combined with small amounts of meat are good sources of protein and can be used to extend meat dishes for economy.

Fruit Exchanges

1. Use a variety of fruits and try them as appetizers, with a main course, or as a dessert.

2. Avoid both canned and frozen fruit that have sugar added. Both water-packed canned fruits and sugar-free frozen fruits are surprisingly flavorful and sweet. For economical reasons, canned fruits are sometimes the most sensible buy. If water-packed fruits are not available, choose fruits preserved in a light syrup, rinse the syrup from the fruit before using and count as 1 fruit exchange and 1 miscellaneous food exchange.

3. Canned fruit juices should be purchased without added sugar. This requires reading the labels on the cans carefully.

Vegetable Exchanges

1. Cook vegetables in a small amount of rapidly boiling water until just tender in order to retain flavor, nutrient content, and a pleasing texture. Save the liquid for soups. Try boiling in bouillon, or steam or bake vegetables for variety.

2. Peel only a thin layer of skin when preparing vegetables to retain the nutrients found right under the skin. Scrub young vegetables instead of peeling.

3. Experiment with herbs, spices, seasoned salts, vinegar, or lemon juice for added flavor.

4. Try interesting combinations of cooked vegetables such as cauliflower and peas, peppers and onions, or broccoli and mushrooms.

5. Use combinations of raw vegetables as salads, snacks, and appetizers. Try vegetables that are not usually served raw, such as cauliflower and mushrooms. Add salt or herbed vinegar for flavor. Use vegetable dips of herbed whipped cottage cheese with raw vegetables for an occasional hors d'oeuvre treat. Raw vegetables, due to their bulk, are eaten in less quantity than when cooked. They are considered calorie-free foods and do not need to be recorded on the daily food plan.

Milk Exchanges

1. Use milk products that have had the milk fat removed (skimmed milk), for the caloric value is halved. Because the fat-soluble vitamin A is removed with the milk fat, buy skimmed milk fortified with both vitamins D and A. Both fluid and dry skim milk can be fortified. The use of dried skim milk powder in cooking and as a beverage is an

economical measure. If mixed well in advance and allowed to become thoroughly chilled, the flavor is comparable to fluid skimmed milk.

2. Milk exchanges may also be used in soups, eggnogs, custards, and on cereals.

3. Find recipes that substitute low-calorie milk products for the calorie-rich creams commonly used in desserts, toppings, and dips. Whipped evaporated skimmed milk can replace whipped creams in some desserts; whipped cottage cheese or yogurt can replace sour cream or mayonnaise in salad and fruit dressings and dips; and flavored skim milk powder can be whipped and used instead of whipped cream.

4. Try plain yogurt and unsweetened fruit, or plain yogurt sprinkled lightly with brown sugar and cinnamon. The calorie value of commercially flavored yogurt will vary with the brand but in general will be twice as high as plain yogurt.

5. Ice milk is a good source of calcium and is included on the milk exchange list. Choose it in preference to ice cream and measure amounts carefully.

Miscellaneous Foods

1. Fat has over twice as many calories per gram as carbohydrates or protein. Measure accurately when using butter, margarine, and oils.

2. Margarines and vegetable oils contain polyunsaturated fatty acids which are a dietary essential. It is wise not to completely exclude such foods from a diet.

3. Low-calorie cookbooks have a variety of suggestions for salad dressings.

4. When choosing wine as a beverage, use light dry wines instead of the more caloric sweet heavy ones.

5. Use club soda, water, or ice as a mixer with alcoholic beverages.

6. On social occasions substitute low-calorie beverages for alcoholic drinks but drink them from regular wine, cocktail, or liquor glasses.

7. Avoid all the high-calorie appetizers that frequently accompany alcoholic beverages.

8. Some low-calorie desserts, such as angel food cake, jello, and sherbet, have been included on the miscellaneous exchange list. Other desserts may be found in low-calorie cookbooks and may be used as well, but such desserts should not supply more than 80 calories per serving. They may be used alone or combined with fruits.

Foods with negligible calories

1. Experiment with herbs, spices, vinegars, and seasonings to add flavor and interest to foods.

2. Use hot herbed teas, iced tea, coffee, decaffeinated coffee, and hot bouillons when you are not really hungry but feel like eating or drinking something.

3. Limited amounts of sugar substitutes may be used as flavoring. Recent research has indicated saccharin to be noncarcinogenic[25] and it has been included on the calorie-free list. However it is not recommended that any sugar substitute be used indiscriminately, as reconditioning of the desire for concentrated sweets is needed. Besides, little is known about the long-term effects of such substitutes. For the same reason, the drinking of diet pop should be limited, and it is always necessary to read the labels of these beverages for caloric content. They may have to be counted as one or more miscellaneous exchanges.

4. Keep a selection of raw vegetables prepared in airtight containers in the refrigerator so they are handy for snacks. It is important that they be prepared beforehand and available immediately in order to resist the temptation of instant high-calorie snack foods.

SUMMARY

The diet management program consists of the following steps:

1. The choice of a caloric level to maintain an average loss of one pound of body fat per week through dietary restriction.

2. The choice of a food plan based on food exchanges to provide approximately this number of calories.

3. The daily recording of food eaten on the provided vinyl folder.

4. The daily graphing of this intake on the provided Eating-Weight-Exercise graph.

Concurrent with these steps, the preparation of food so as to control caloric content yet maintain interest and flavor is essential.

If the mechanics of the diet management program—the exchange list system and individualized daily food plan—are understood, the use of the exchange foods and the record-keeping system are simply and quickly accomplished and facilitate adherence to diet reconditioning and weight loss. A programmed learning section follows in order to help the dieter become more familiar with this system. It is recommended that this program be completed before beginning the diet regimen.

Programmed Learning Section

Each page in this section has two columns. The left column gives information followed by a question or questions. A space is left after the question to write in the answer. The right column gives the answers to the questions. These answers should be kept covered until after the question has been answered *in writing*. Much of the information required to answer the questions will be found on the food exchange lists in Appendix C. These lists and the instructions with them should be read before beginning the program.

For each question, therefore:

1. Make sure the answer column is covered;
2. Read the information given;
3. Read the question and then write the answer in the allotted space;
4. Compare your answer with the one in the answer column.

1. An energy deficit of approximately 3,500 calories will result in the use of one pound of body fat for energy. This deficit may be established through a decrease in caloric intake, an increase in energy expenditure, or a combination of the two.

Question 1a:
If you wish to lose one pound of body fat in a week, your total *weekly* food intake must be _____ calories *less* than you actually need.

Answer 1a:
3,500

Question 1b:
If you wish to lose one pound of body fat in a week, your total *daily* food intake must be _____ calories *less* than what you actually need.

Answer 1b:
500

Question 1c:
Cycling rapidly will use approximately 500 calories of energy in one hour. If you added a brisk hour's bicycle ride to your daily activities and kept your food intake constant, how much body fat would you use up in one week? _____

Answer 1c:
1 pound

If you decreased your daily caloric intake by 500 calories and added an hour's strenuous bicycle riding to your daily schedule, how much body weight would you lose in one week? _____

Answer 1d:
2 pounds

2. Caloric requirements are affected by activity level, age, size, and sex. Refer to Table 1, Chapter 5 on page 139 to find the approximate daily caloric needs for your age and sex and for a light level of physical activity. This is only an approximation, as your body size will also affect your caloric needs.

Question 2a:
For your age and sex, approximately how many calories do you require per day?

_____

Answer 2a:
See Table 1,
Chapter 5

Question 2b:
If you require approximately 2,000 calories per day, how many calories would it be necessary for you to eat per day in order to lose one pound of fat per week, providing that your energy expenditure remains constant? _____

Answer 2b:
1,500

3. A weight reduction diet should provide foods that supply essential nutrients. Food exchange lists offer a selection of dairy foods, meats, breads, cereals, vegetables, fruits, and miscellaneous foods which allow a diet balanced in all essential nutrients. A list of foods that provide only negligible calories, called calorie-free foods, is also included.

Question 3a:
Refer to the food exchange lists and write the six types of exchanges allowed on your diet, giving an example of each.

	FOOD GROUP	EXAMPLE
1.	_____	_____
2.	_____	_____
3.	_____	_____
4.	_____	_____
5.	_____	_____
6.	_____	_____

Answer 3a:
FOOD GROUPS:
Meats
Cereals
Milk
Vegetables
Fruits
Miscellaneous
EXAMPLES:
See exchange lists

4. Each food on the same list, in the amount specified, is similar in caloric value and is called an exchange because it may be exchanged or substituted for any other food on that same list. For example, either a small potato, a slice of bread, or 1/2 cup of cooked macaroni noodles may be used whenever a cereal exchange is allowed on the food plan.

Question 4a:

Read the exchange lists carefully and then write the list on which each of the following foods is found.

1. Eggs _____
2. Peanut butter _____
3. Yogurt _____
4. Cooked cereal _____
5. Raisins _____
6. Tomatoes _____
7. Mushrooms _____
8. Sauerkraut _____
9. Syrup _____
10. Macaroni noodles _____
11. Corn on the cob _____
12. Angel food cake _____
13. Frankfurter _____
14. Mayonnaise _____
15. Bacon _____
16. Wine _____

Answer 4a:
1. Meat
2. Meat
3. Milk
4. Cereal
5. Fruit
6. Fruit
7. Vegetable
8. Vegetable
9. Miscellaneous
10. Cereal
11. Cereal
12. Miscellaneous
13. Meat
14. Miscellaneous
15. Miscellaneous
16. Miscellaneous

5. Each meat exchange supplies approximately 75 calories. Meats and meat products vary in fat content, and the use of

the low-fat meat exchanges is encouraged. An average serving portion of *cooked* meat, poultry, or fish at dinner generally weighs 3 to 5 ounces. It is important that the weights of serving portions are accurate, as people tend to differ markedly in their estimates of portion size of meats. Exchanges are always based on the weight of meat *after cooking.*

Question 5a:
If you choose 3 ounces of veal for dinner, how many meat exchanges have you used?
_____

Answer 5a:
3

Question 5b:
If you choose 1 egg and 1 ounce of ham for breakfast, how many meat exchanges have you used? _____

Answer 5b:
2

Question 5c:
If you make a salad using 1/2 cup of tuna fish and 1 ounce of diced cheddar cheese, how many meat exchanges have you used?
_____

Answer 5c:
3

6. Foods listed on the cereal exchange list supply approximately 70 calories of energy. The use of whole grain and enriched breads and cereals, crackers, and pastas is recommended. Starchy vegetables and soups are also included on the cereal exchange list.

Question 6a:
List the vegetables included on the cereal exchange list. Specify the amounts to equal 1 cereal exchange.

_____
_____
_____
_____
_____
_____

Answer 6a:

Potato (1 small or
   ½ cup mashed)
Corn (1 ear or ½ cup)
Parsnips (½ cup)
Dried beans and peas
   (½ cup)
Sweet potatoes (¼ cup)
Baked beans in
   sauce (¼ cup)

7. Each milk exchange supplies approximately 85 calories. Most of the milk exchanges are based on skimmed or partially skimmed milk, as whole milk has twice the caloric value of fat-free milk.

Question 7a:
Give the amounts of the following foods that equal 1 milk exchange:
1. Buttermilk (made from skimmed milk)
   _____

2. Plain yogurt (made from partially skimmed milk—2%) _____
3. Ice milk
4. Cottage cheese (plain) _____

Answer 7a:
1. 1 cup
2. 3/4 cup
3. 1/3 cup
4. 1/2 cup

8. Vegetables vary somewhat in carbohydrate content and therefore they have been divided into two groups. The vegetables of the first group supply negligible amounts of carbohydrates, and you may use up to 1 cup of cooked vegetables to equal 1 vegetable exchange. The vegetables of the second section contain somewhat more carbohydrates, and it is recommended that you *average* each day *one* 1/2 cup serving (cooked) of these higher carbohydrate vegetables. A total of 3 exchanges from the vegetable exchange list (2 from List 1 and 1 from List 2) supply approximately 50 calories in all.

Question 8a:
Which of the following vegetables are found on the vegetable exchange list? For each of these specify the amounts of *cooked* vegetables that are equal to one vegetable exchange.
1. Cabbage _____
2. Carrots _____
3. Tomatoes _____
4. Peas _____

Answer 8a:
1. Up to 1 cup
2. ½ cup
3. See fruit exchange list
4. ½ cup

5. Parsnips _____	5. See cereal exchange list
6. Sauerkraut _____	6. Up to 1 cup
7. Corn _____	7. See cereal exchange list
8. Spinach _____	8. Up to 1 cup
9. Green beans _____	9. Up to 1 cup

9. Most vegetables commonly eaten raw are negligible in caloric value, and you are allowed to eat them in reasonable amounts when desired. Both carrots and turnips are slightly higher in carbohydrate content, however because you are encouraged to eat a variety of raw vegetables, *all raw* vegetables are counted as free foods.

Question 9a:
List vegetables on the vegetable exchange lists that may be eaten raw:

_____
_____
_____
_____
_____
_____
_____
_____
_____
_____
_____
_____
_____
_____

Answer 9a:
The following are possibilities, but answers will vary according to individual tastes.

Cabbage
Carrots
Cauliflower
Celery
Cucumbers
Endive
Green beans, young
Green onions
Greens
Lettuce
Mushrooms
Peppers
Radishes
Turnips
Watercress

10. Fruits on the fruit exchange list, in the amounts specified, supply approximately 40 calories per exchange. They may be eaten raw or cooked as long as no sugar has been added. It is necessary to carefully read the labels of cans and packages of fruits and fruit juices to make sure they do not contain additional sugar.

Question 10a:

Specify the amounts of the following fruits to equal 1 fruit exchange, and check those rich in vitamin C.

1. Apple juice _____
2. Strawberries _____
3. Tomato juice _____
4. Banana _____
5. Applesauce _____
6. Cantaloupe _____
7. Raisins _____
8. Grapefruit _____

Answer 10a:
1. ½ cup
2. 1 cup
3. 1 cup
4. ½ small
5. ½ cup
6. ¼ small
7. 2 tablespoons
8. ½ small

11. The foods listed on the miscellaneous list supply concentrated sources of calories. They should be used sparingly.

Question 11a:

If 1 teaspoon of vegetable oil is used in salad dressing, how many miscellaneous exchanges would be recorded? _____

Answer 11a:
1

Question 11b:

If 3 ounces of dry wine were chosen to drink with a meal, how many miscellaneous food exchanges would be recorded on the daily food plan? _____

Answer 11b:
2

Question 11c:

A beverage consisting of 1 jigger (1½ ounces) of rye mixed with water would use how many miscellaneous food exchanges?

_____

Answer 11c:
3

12. The foods and food items that have negligible caloric value may be used as desired and do not have to be recorded on the daily food plan. The use of these will not significantly affect the caloric value of your diet, and they are excellent as flavoring substances, appetizers, and snacks.

Question 12a:
List the beverages allowed on the free-calorie foods list:

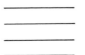

Answer 12a:
Bouillon
Broths, clear
Coffee
Tea

13. The use of food exchanges is a quick and easy method for controlling daily calorie levels. Each day you are allowed a certain number of exchanges from each of the exchange lists to make up your daily food plan. From your daily allotment of exchanges you may choose the specific foods you wish to eat at each meal. At each meal it is essential that you record the number and kind of exchanges you have eaten by writing the *time* of eating on your daily food plan. This ensures a constant reminder of the number of exchanges remaining of your daily allotment as well as food distribution throughout the day. The following questions will give you some practice in planning meals using food exchanges.

Question 13a:
You have chosen for breakfast 1 cup (8 ounces) of tomato juice, 1 ounce of broiled ham, 2 pieces of toast with margarine (1 teaspoon) and honey (1 tablespoon), and a cup of black coffee. Use a check mark to indicate the exchanges you would record on your daily food plan.

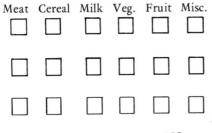

Meat Cereal Milk Veg. Fruit Misc.

Answer 13a:
1 Meat (ham)
2 Cereal (2 pieces toast)
1 Fruit
2 Miscellaneous (margarine, honey)

159

Question 13b:

For lunch you have chosen 1 bowl of onion soup (1/3 can diluted with water), a crab salad (using 1/2 cup of crab, lettuce, cucumber, celery, and lemon juice), a roll with 1 teaspoon margarine, a sliced apple with cinnamon, and iced tea. Check the exchanges you would record on your daily food plan.

Meat Cereal Milk Veg. Fruit Misc.

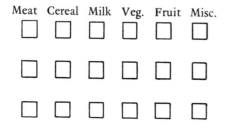

Answer 13b:
2 Meat (2 ounces crab)
2 Cereal (muffin,
    onion soup)
1 Fruit (apple)
1 Miscellaneous
    (Margarine)

Question 13c:

For dinner you have chosen a tossed salad of raw vegetables with an herbed vinegar dressing, 3 ounces baked chicken, 1/2 cup cooked carrots, and a combination of 1 cup broccoli and 1/2 cup cauliflower flavored with herbs. For dessert you have chosen a cup of fresh strawberries with 1/3 cup of ice milk and black coffee. Check the exchanges you would use for this meal.

Meat Cereal Milk Veg. Fruit Misc.

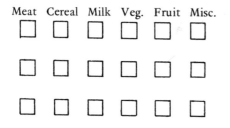

Answer 13c:
3 Meat (chicken)
1 Milk (ice milk)
3 Vegetable (carrots,
    broccoli, cauliflower)
1 Fruit (strawberries)

Question 13d:

By adding the caloric values of each exchange, calculate the caloric value of the dinner in Question 13c. _____

Answer 13d:
3 Meat	225
1 Milk	85
3 Vegetables	50
1 Fruit	40
	400

Question 13e:

For a bedtime snack you have chosen 1 cup of hot chocolate using 1 cup of skimmed milk and 1 teaspoon (heaping) of sweetened cocoa powder. Check the number and type of exchanges you would use for this snack.

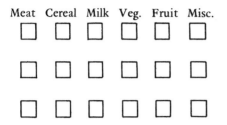

Meat Cereal Milk Veg. Fruit Misc.

Answer 13e:
1 Milk
1 Miscellaneous

14. Recipes for salads, casseroles, and desserts can be prepared using the food exchange system. The following questions will give you some suggestions for using exchanges in a variety of recipes.

Question 14a:

You have prepared spaghetti for dinner. Your serving portion contains 1/2 cup cooked spaghetti noodles with a meat sauce composed of 1/4 cup tomato sauce, onion flakes, chopped garlic, seasonings, and 2 ounces of lean ground beef. Check the kind and number of exchanges you would enter on your daily food plan.

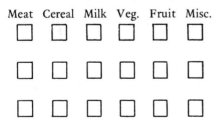

Meat Cereal Milk Veg. Fruit Misc.

Answer 14a:
2 Meat (2 ounces ground beef)
2 Cereal (noodles, tomato sauce)

Question 14b:

You have prepared baked chicken with pineapple and rice for dinner. Your serving portion consists of 3 ounces chicken, chicken broth, 1 cup sliced peppers and mushrooms, 1/2 cup of pineapple pieces, seasonings, and 1/2 cup of parsleyed rice. Check the kind and number of exchanges you would enter on your daily food plan.

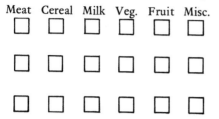

Answer 14b:
3 Meat (3 ounces chicken)
1 Cereal (rice)
1 Vegetable (peppers and mushrooms)
1 Fruit (pineapple)

Question 14c:

You have prepared baked apple crunch for dessert. The recipe calls for 1 sliced apple, lemon juice, cinnamon, 1 heaping teaspoon brown sugar with a topping of 2 graham crackers (each 2½ inches square) and 1 teaspoon melted margarine. Check the number and kinds of food exchanges used in this recipe.

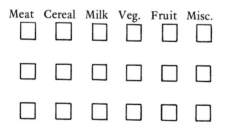

Answer 14c:
1 Cereal (crackers)
1 Fruit (apple)
2 Miscellaneous (brown sugar, margarine)

FOOTNOTES

1. Shakespeare, W. Hamlet, Prince of Denmark. In R. G. White (Ed.), *The Riverside Shakespeare*. Vol. VI. *Tragedies*. Boston: Houghton, Mifflin, 1883. P. 523.
2. Hodges, R. E. Present knowledge of carbohydrates. In *Present knowledge in nutrition*. New York: The Nutrition Foundation, 1967.
3. Yudkin, J. The treatment of obesity by the "high-fat" diet: The inevitability of calories. *The Lancet*, 1960, *2*, 939-941.
4. Pilkington, T. R. E., Gainsborough, H., Rosenoer, V. M., and Carey, I. Diet and weight-reduction in the obese. *The Lancet*, 1960, *1*, 856-858; Olesen, E. S. and Quaade, F. Fatty foods and obesity. *The Lancet*, 1960, *1*, 1048-1051; and Bortz, W. M., Wroldsen, A., and Morris, P. Effects of salt on rate of weight loss with isocaloric substitutions of carbohydrate and fat. *Federation Proceedings*, 1967, *26*, 473.
5. Yudkin, J. Doctors' treatment of obesity, analysis of the Practitioner Questionnaire. *Practitioner*, 1968, *201*, 330-335.
6. Bloom, W. L. and Azar, G. J. Similarities of carbohydrate deficiency and fasting. *Archives of Internal Medicine*, 1963, *112*, 333-343.
7. National Research Council, Food and Nutrition Board. *Recommended Dietary Allowances*. (Publication 1694, 7th rev. ed.) Washington, D.C.: National Academy of Sciences, 1968.
8. Davidson, S. and Passmore, R. *Human nutrition and dietetics*. Edinburgh: E. and S. Livingstone, 1969.
9. Pike, R. L. and Brown, M. L. *Nutrition: An integrated approach*. New York: John Wiley, 1967.
10. Mayer, J. *Overweight: Causes, cost and control*. Englewood Cliffs, N. J.: Prentice-Hall, 1968.
11. Hartsook, E. W. and Hershberger, T. V. Influence of low, intermediate, and high levels of dietary protein on heat production of rats. *Journal of Nutrition*, 1963, *81*, 209-217.
12. Griffith, W. H. and Dyer, H. M. Present knowledge of specific dynamic action. In *Present knowledge in nutrition, op. cit.*
13. Davidson and Passmore, *op. cit.*
14. Turner, D. *Handbook of diet therapy*. Chicago: University of Chicago Press, 1965.
15. National Research Council, Committee on Food Habits. *The problem of changing food habits: Report of the Committee on Food Habits 1941-1943*. (Bulletin 108) Washington, D.C.: National Academy of Sciences, 1943.
16. Burgess, A. and Dean, R. F. A. *Malnutrition and food habits*. London: Tavistock, 1962; and Wenkam, N. S. Cultural determinants of nutritional behavior. *Nutrition Program News* (U. S. Department of Agriculture, Washington, D.C.), July-August 1969.
17. Young, C. M., Moore, N. S., Berresford, K., Einset, B. M., and Waldner, B. G. The problem of the obese patient. *Journal of the American Dietetic Association*, 1955, *31*, 1111-1115.
18. Bortz, W. M. Predictability of weight loss. *Journal of the American Medical Association*, 1968, *204*, 101-105.
19. Bray, G. A. Effect of caloric restriction on energy expenditure in obese patients. *The Lancet*, 1969, *2*, 397-398.
20. Mayer, *op. cit.*
21. Bortz, *op. cit.*
22. Turner, *op. cit.*
23. Stunkard, A. J., Grace, W. J., and Wolff, H. G. The night eating syndrome—a pattern of food intake among certain obese patients. *American Journal of Medicine*, 1955, *19*, 78-85.
24. Metabolic changes in "meal-fed" rats. *Nutrition Reviews*, 1970, *28*, 234-235.
25. Study reveals saccharin does not cause cancer. *Food Technology*, 1970, *24*, 46.

Chapter 6

PHYSICAL ACTIVITY: A FACTOR IN WEIGHT CONTROL AND GENERAL HEALTH

The third aspect of the threefold treatment of obesity is physical activity. Many of the chronic and degenerative diseases afflicting modern societies appear to result from the living habits of the individual within these societies, and physical activity and sound nutrition are primary preventive measures. Dr. Hans Kraus has coined the term hypokinetic diseases (i.e., caused by insufficient motion) to describe the whole spectrum of disorders that may be influenced or induced by physical inactivity,[1] and obesity would definitely have to be included.

COMMON MISCONCEPTIONS REGARDING PHYSICAL ACTIVITY

Traditionally, physical activity has been ignored or discredited in weight control owing to two misconceptions regarding the role of exercise and the control of body weight. It is commonly believed, first, that exercise plays an insignificant role in total body energy requirements and that increases in exertion will not appreciably increase the body's calorie requirements and, second, that increases in exercise always result in increased appetite, hence in increased food consumption. It is worthwhile to examine both of these concepts in more detail.

Physical activity as part of the total energy requirements. The total energy requirement of the body includes the energy needed to carry on vital function and nutrient utilization while the body is at complete rest, as well as the energy required for physical exertion. Vital function includes the beating of the heart, breathing, maintenance of muscle tone, movement of compounds in and out of the body cells, maintenance of body temperature, and a host of other activities. The energy needed to maintain these functions is called basal energy. The rate at which an individual uses energy to satisfy basal needs is called the basal metabolic rate and is measured in calories per square meter of body surface per hour. This rate varies with age, size, and sex. It is highest in actively growing young children, due to the energy needed for tissue growth, and declines slowly through adulthood (see Figure 1). This decline in energy need associated with continued high-calorie intake perhaps contributes to the "middle age spread" of the average American.[2] In addition to age, size affects basal needs—the smaller person having a somewhat lower basal metabolic rate than the larger. Sex is a third influence, with women having a basal metabolic rate approximately 6 to 7 percent lower than men of the same size and age.[3] Table 1 shows basal caloric requirements per day for both men and women of varying sizes. These basal requirements are a considerable proportion of total energy needs, particularly in sedentary individuals. It has frequently been suggested that obese people have lower basal needs than their more slender counterparts and that this has led to their obese state. Studies on obese people, however, do not substantiate this, as their basal metabolic rates appear to be within normal ranges.[4] Research to date has not discovered any dependable differences in basal energy needs that lead to the development of obesity.

In addition to the energy needed for maintenance of vital function, a small increment is needed for the utilization of food nutrients. This has been described in the previous chapter as the specific dynamic action (SDA) of food. With a mixed diet containing carbohydrates, fats, and

FIGURE 1

CHANGES IN BASAL METABOLIC RATES WITH AGE

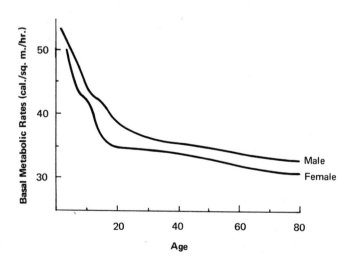

TABLE 1
BASAL METABOLIC REQUIREMENTS
FOR VARIOUS NORMAL BODY WEIGHTS

Body weight (lb.)	Basal metabolic requirement (age 22)
Men	
154	1690
165	1770
176	1820
187	1900
198	1990
209	2060
220	2140
Women	
99	1240
110	1310
121	1400
128	1460
132	1480
143	1570
154	1650

Adapted from National Research Council, Food and Nutrition Board, *Recommended Dietary Allowances.* (Publication 1694 7th rev. ed.) Washington, D.C.: National Academy of Sciences, 1968. P. 5.

protein the specific dynamic effect of food results in an approximate 6 percent increase in energy expenditure over the basal amount. This is but a small portion of total energy expenditure.

Physical activity is the third factor influencing total energy requirement and includes the energy to support the body while sitting and standing as well as energy to move the body while walking, running, lifting, climbing, carrying, etc. These costs must be added to the resting requirement in order to calculate total energy needs. The needs for physical activity may vary markedly due to occupational differences, recreational activities, and individual variation, however like individuals appear to be quite similar in their caloric needs for basal function and food utilization.[5] Thus physical exertion is the most variable factor determining the total energy requirement. Inactive individuals may require a caloric

FIGURE 2
**DIAGRAMMATIC REPRESENTATION ILLUSTRATING
THE EFFECTS OF PHYSICAL ACTIVITY ON TOTAL ENERGY NEEDS**

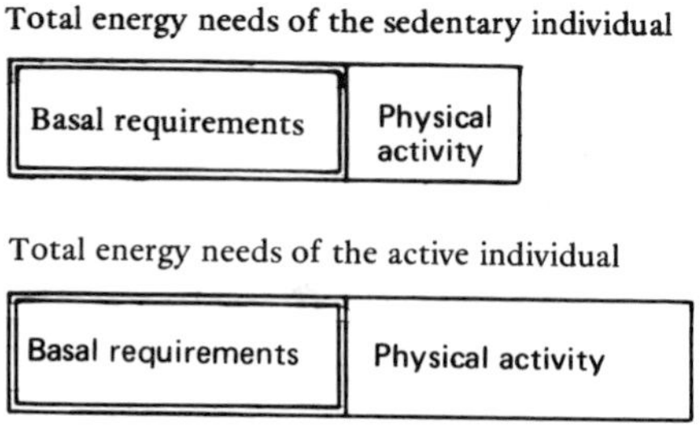

Total energy needs of the sedentary individual

Basal requirements	Physical activity

Total energy needs of the active individual

Basal requirements	Physical activity

increase of only 40 to 50 percent above their basal needs to satisfy the total energy requirement, whereas strenuously active persons may need increases of 100 percent or more above basal needs (see Figure 2).[6] The variations in daily energy expenditure of men working in a variety of occupations are shown in Table 2. The mean calorie expenditure range of 2,330 to 3,670 from the least active to the most active group illustrates the effect of physical activity in determining the calorie needs of individuals and reinforces the fact that physical exertion may indeed increase total caloric requirements considerably.

Physical activity and food intake. The belief that an increase in activity levels will always increase appetite and therefore food intake has been a part of many past and present weight-control regimens, however research suggests that this is not necessarily the case. Intricate physiological mechanisms act to balance food intake with energy expenditure, but research with both animals and humans suggests that these mechanisms only work adequately within *normal* ranges of physical activity.[7] It appears that animals require certain critical levels of activity for normal regulation of the intricately operating appetite-regulatory mechanisms. Farmers have long been aware of the fact that animals will not restrict their food intake to balance extremely low levels of activity, and hence they curtail the activity of animals they wish to fatten for market—a practice known as penning or cooping. Similar results can be seen with pets restricted to the house.

In the same manner, the extremely low levels of human activity that are possible in modern industrialized societies do not, perhaps, allow normal regulation of intake with expenditure. Actually, it has been shown that at a truly sedentary level food intake may actually increase slightly.[8]

TABLE 2

**DAILY RATES OF ENERGY EXPENDITURE BY
INDIVIDUALS WITH VARIOUS OCCUPATIONS**

| Occupation | Energy expenditure (kcal/day) | | |
	Mean	Minimum	Maximum
Elderly retired	2330	1750	2810
Office workers	2520	1820	3270
Colliery clerks	2800	2330	3290
Laboratory technicians	2840	2240	3820
Elderly industrial workers	2840	2180	3710
University students	2930	2270	4410
Building workers	3000	2440	3730
Steel workers	3280	2600	3960
Army cadets	3490	2990	4100
Elderly peasants (Swiss)	3530	2210	5000
Farmers	3550	2450	4670
Coal miners	3660	2970	4560
Forestry workers	3670	2860	4600

Reproduced with permission from J. V. G. A. Durnin and R. Passmore, *Energy, work and leisure.* London: Heinemann Educational Books Ltd., 1967. Pp. 115-116.

A change in activity patterns, therefore, from a sedentary level to a moderate level will not necessarily stimulate appetite so as to cancel out the benefit of the added energy expenditure, but may in fact contribute to a reduction in food intake.

The curvilinear relation between food intake and energy expenditure among adults in different occupational groups is illustrated in Figure 3. Based upon the research of Jean Mayer, the data summarized in this figure demonstrate that food intake actually declines as movement is made from low- to moderate-activity occupations, rising as a function of increased energy demands associated with work after that point. Furthermore, the effect of food intake and levels of exertion on body weight are illustrated in Figure 4. If these data derived from group observations can be extended to individuals, they would suggest that for each person a critical point might be reached at which food consumption would be at its low point relative to energy expenditure. Few people should allow their exertion level to fall below this critical point.

As well as allowing long-term normal functioning of appetite-control mechanisms, exercise may affect food intake in other respects. Strenuous exercise before a meal frequently acts to decrease appetite for that meal.

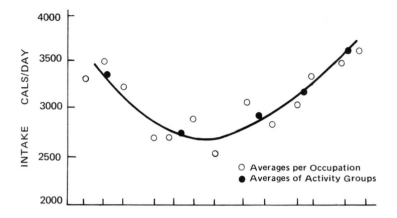

FIGURES 3 and 4
CALORIC INTAKE AS A
FUNCTION OF PHYSICAL ACTIVITY

O Averages per Occupation
● Averages of Activity Groups

BODY WEIGHT AS A
FUNCTION OF PHYSICAL ACTIVITY

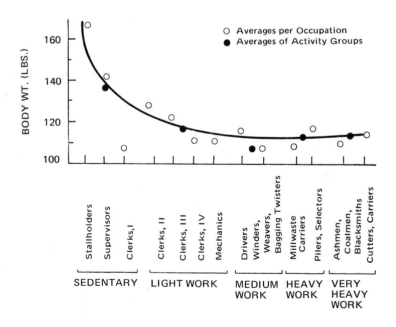

O Averages per Occupation
● Averages of Activity Groups

Reproduced with permission from J. Mayer and B. Bullen, Nutrition and athletic performance. *Physiological Reviews*, 1960. *40*, 374.

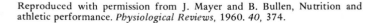

In addition, by adding periods of some form of regular, enjoyable exertion to the daily routine the tension and boredom that frequently stimulate eating may be alleviated. Providing the exercise is pleasurable and ranks higher in the hierarchy of preferred activities than eating, it may serve to replace inappropriate eating.

PHYSICAL ACTIVITY IN THE ETIOLOGY, TREATMENT, AND PREVENTION OF OBESITY

From the information presented in the preceding section, it is evident that physical activity can exert a considerable influence on the energy needs of the body and that certain amounts of exertion may be required for a normally functioning appetite. Furthermore, much evidence implicates inactivity as a contributing factor to obesity.

Inactivity as a factor contributing to obesity. The creeping overweight or "middle age spread" that is common in industrialized societies but not in developing countries can perhaps be attributed to a decrease in physical activity as well as the slow decline in basal metabolism. A study of the leisure-time activity patterns of males living in Tecumseh, Michigan, illustrates this pattern of decreasing physical exertion with age. A total of 1,695 subjects, aged 16 to 69, were included in this study. In general, the time spent in active leisure decreased with each older age group (see Table 3).[9]

Observations of the patterns of eating and physical activity in large populations also indicate a causal role for inactivity. National averages of caloric intake indicate that Americans are consuming *slightly fewer* calories than their predecessors.[10] Mechanization, however, has *markedly* decreased the need for physical exertion, and people are exercising considerably less than their forebearers. When viewing the national picture it would seem that, *on the whole,* Americans are perhaps not overindulging but merely overeating for their energy needs. In fact, researchers over thirty years ago were questioning the emphasis traditionally placed on "whether the fat man eats much or little" and were instead stressing the importance of the relationship between consumption and activity.[11]

Investigations of the activity patterns of some obese individuals also raise the question of inactivity as a contributing factor, as low levels of exertion have been demonstrated in comparison with the levels of normal-weight persons. Studies with obese and normal-weight adolescent girls showed that the majority of obese girls actually ate slightly less than the normal-weight girls but also exercised considerably less.[12] Investigations with adolescent boys yielded similar but less striking results.[13]

TABLE 3
FREQUENCY DISTRIBUTION OF NUMBER OF HOURS PARTICIPATION IN LEISURE TIME ACTIVITIES BY AGE

Hours of Activity[a]	% Participation by Age (Yrs.)					All Ages
	16-29	30-39	40-49	50-59	60-69	
0	1.9	1.8	3.2	5.4	9.4	3.4
0.1-0.9	8.6	8.9	12.3	16.1	19.5	11.7
1.0-1.9	17.5	16.4	21.6	18.8	15.4	18.2
2.0-4.9	36.9	39.9	36.0	38.3	31.5	37.3
5.0-9.9	23.6	25.7	19.7	16.9	20.8	21.9
10+	11.4	7.3	7.2	4.6	3.4	7.4
N	360	494	431	261	149	1695

a. Hours of active leisure time activities per week pro-rated for one year.

Reproduced with permission from D. A. Cunningham, H. J. Montoye, H. L. Metzner, and J. B. Keller, Active leisure time activities as related to age among males in a total population. *Journal of Gerontology*, 1968, *23*, 552.

Another study using time motion pictures of obese and normal-weight girls found that obese girls expended less energy than the nonobese subjects even though both groups were involved in the *same* scheduled activity (see Figure 5).[14] Furthermore, studies on adults demonstrated that obese men and women walked less than normal-weight controls who lived in the same area and were involved in similar occupations. The distance walked was measured with pedometers which, while not yielding precise values on total energy expenditure, are nevertheless useful for rough comparisons. As Table 4 shows, there was a difference in the number of miles walked per day between the two groups,[15] with the contrast between the obese and nonobese women being the most marked.

In light of these findings, the question must be considered as to what extent the decreased activity is a product of or a contribution to the obese state. If not a causal factor, inactivity is undoubtedly perpetuating the condition, and it is clear that patterns of activity as well as eating habits must be considered in treatment programs.

Physical activity—its role in weight reduction. A role for exercise in weight reduction has frequently been belittled. It has been stated, for example, that one must climb the stairs to the top of the Empire State Building and down again repeatedly for four hours in order to lose one pound of body fat. Such statistics would dampen the enthusiasm of the most ardent devotee of exercise. However, it is also true that if that same individual climbed the stairs to his fourth-floor office and back down again four times a day, he would lose that pound of fat in thirty days or six working weeks. This would result in a yearly loss of approximately nine pounds. Those who wish to negate the role of exercise describe any exhausting task as taking place for prolonged uninterrupted periods of time for it to be effective. This is not necessary. Short but regular periods of exercise will make the same contribution and can be a useful and enjoyable adjunct to weight-reduction regimens.

Carefully controlled studies on small groups of people have demonstrated that when diet and exercise are combined, regular exercise increases the rate of weight loss. Furthermore, it is well-known that the obese individual will burn more calories per minute than his lean

FIGURE 5
PERCENT OF OBESE AND NONOBESE GIRLS
INACTIVE DURING SPORTS

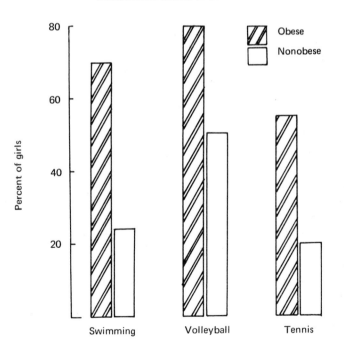

Adapted from B. Bullen, R. B. Reed, and J. Mayer, Physical activity of obese and nonobese adolescent girls appraised by motion picture sampling. *American Journal of Clinical Nutrition,* 1964. *14,* 217.

TABLE 4

**SUMMARY OF DATA ON OVERWEIGHT
IN RELATION TO MILES WALKED**

Group	Median Amount Overweight %	Mean Age yr.	Mean Daily Distance Walked (mi.)	P Value
Men:				
Obese	54	36	3.7±1.8	< 0.05
Nonobese		36½	6.0±4.3	
Women:				
Obese	52	42	2.0±1.2	<0.01
Nonobese		40	4.9±2.1	

Reproduced with permission from A. M. Chirico and A. J. Stunkard, Physical activity and human obesity. *New England Journal of Medicine*, 1960, *263*, 937.

counterpart when carrying out the same task. Thus, while dietary restriction has the most dramatic effect on weight reduction regular exercise can in the long run make a contribution. A study of obese college women demonstrated an approximate 10 percent increase in weight loss when four exercise periods a week were coupled with dietary restriction; moreover, the investigators reported better control of fluid retention and a more positive mental attitude among the exercising subjects.[16] Another study reported increased rate of weight loss when regular periods of walking were included in the reduction regimen.[17] Interestingly, the salutary effect of exercise was most pronounced when caloric restriction was not excessive, and the decreased effectiveness was suspected to result from metabolic compensation to severe caloric restriction. Exercise alone has also been shown to result in weight reduction. Two groups of sedentary middle-aged males taking part in a two-year study demonstrated that those exercising reduced weight and increased fitness as well, while their nonexercising counterparts showed weight gains during the same period.[18]

Exercise has yet another benefit to the dieter: By increasing energy expenditure it is not necessary to restrict caloric intake severely in order to yield encouraging results. The deprivation and hunger that often accompany dieting probably contribute more to an inability to adhere to a regimen than any other factor. By moderately decreasing intake and increasing expenditure, such discomforts can be avoided.

Physical activity as a preventive measure. When considering the failure rate in the treatment of obesity, one might conclude that prevention might be an easier solution to the condition than cure. Regular physical activity is an essential part of preventive measures and undoubtedly is a major factor in the prevention of obesity for many individuals. To quote Jean Mayer: "If we want to avoid obesity, we must either exercise more or feel hungry all our lives." [19]

For those who are inactive, energy needs are comparatively low, and if a desirable body weight is to be maintained, food intake must be rigidly controlled—neither an easy nor perhaps a nutritionally sound undertaking. In recognition of the decreasing patterns of physical activity in America, the Food and Nutrition Board of the National Research Council has, with each revision, consistently reduced its recommended allowance for calories. With the last revision in 1968, however, it was recommended that individuals not reduce their caloric intake below the present allowances and that in order to remain in energy balance and prevent obesity it was preferable to increase expenditure rather than decrease intake further. [20] By increasing exercise, a more relaxed and more satisfying dietary program can be enjoyed, or in the words of Jean Mayer, "regular exercise . . . can be a substitute for regular deprivation." [21]

INACTIVITY AND DISEASE

Beyond its impact upon weight, exertion level is also reflected in resistance to disease. Physical activity has traditionally been considered beneficial for optimum health. The fact that exercise maintains good muscle tone, stimulates circulation, and aids digestion has generally been used to promote it. Another factor in favor of increased physical activity, however, is its action as a tension release. Emotional responses to frustrations, anger, and other stress tend to result in muscle tension. Strenuous exercise releases such tension and hence has a tranquilizing effect. Its effect has been described succinctly as "action absorbs anxiety." [22] Recently, though, research has concentrated on the role of physical exertion as a preventive factor in certain disease conditions and also on the possibility of inactivity as an etiological influence on these diseases.

Of greatest interest is the contribution of inactivity on diseases of the cardiovascular system. Such diseases have been attributed to the living habits of modern man and their occurrence has recently been described as "the greatest sustained epidemic confronting mankind." [23] They are generally characterized by a degeneration of the artery walls, resulting in poor blood supply to vital organs. Atherosclerosis of the coronary arteries leads to coronary heart disease, and similar degenerative processes of the cerebral arteries cause strokes. A 22-year-long epidemiological study of cardiovascular disease among approximately 5,000 residents of Framingham, Massachusetts, recently published results indicating that physical activity may offer a measure of protection, particularly against heart disease. Recent published results of this study state:

> Assessment of the risk of disease, using various indices of habitual energy expenditure, has indicated that sedentary men are more susceptible to coronary attacks than are physically active men. The least active men, comprising fifteen percent of the males in the study, had about three times the risk of those most active physically.[24]

Figure 6 illustrates the morbidity ratio of the men studied, including the ratio of myocardial infarction (heart attack), angina pectoris (disease symptoms), and sudden death.

FIGURE 6

**RISK OF DEVELOPING CORONARY HEART DISEASE
(10 YEARS) ACCORDING TO PHYSICAL ACTIVITY INDEX**

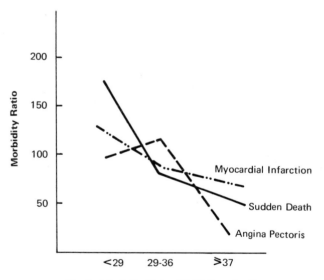

Physical Activity Status At 4th Examination

Reproduced with permission from W. B. Kannel, The disease of living. *Nutrition Today,* 1971, *6 (3),* 5.

How physical activity protects is somewhat a matter of speculation at present. Vigorous physical exercise has been demonstrated to lower the levels of certain fats circulating in the blood.[25] High blood pressure is associated with cardiovascular diseases and physical exercise may exert a helpful effect on this condition.[26] Finally, exercise may exert a direct beneficial effect on the arteries and vessels of the heart as well as developing extra circulation routes or increasing collateral circulation.[27]

The lack of warning signs which accompany both heart attacks and strokes plus the fact that neither the heart nor the brain can be restored to full function once diseased argue for the necessity of preventive measures rather than curative ones. Dr. William Kannel, Director of the Framingham Study, stresses preventive measures rather than "seeking more and better remedies for heart attacks and strokes which have already occurred."[28] At present changes in both diet and exercise patterns seem to be the most logical course of prevention for these diseases, and it is wise to begin preventive measures at an early age.

Just how much physical exercise is needed and how intense it should be are the subjects of investigation at present. Exercise programs have been developed that are especially designed to exercise the cardiovascular system. These programs gradually condition the body through strenuous oxygen-demanding exercises until a satisfactory level of physical fitness or conditioning is achieved. This process is called the training effect. The conditioned body is characterized by a slower heart rate, more efficient oxygen utilization, and increased stamina and endurance. Judging from the soaring bicycle sales in America and the number of sweatsuit-clad suburban joggers, some individuals are undertaking the conditioning process. However, in the Tecumseh study cited previously, very few of the 1,695 men studied participated regularly in leisure-time activities requiring the high levels of energy expenditure required for cardiovascular exercise.[29]

The relationships between sedentary levels of activity and disease will undoubtedly continue to be investigated, and future work may reveal the precise effects of both underactivity and strenuous exercise on body function. At present, however, it is suggested that sedentary individuals would do well to gradually increase energy expenditure in order to maintain a desirable weight, losing weight if necessary, and for good health in general.

MECHANIZATION AND PHYSICAL ACTIVITY

Despite the general need for exercise, modern living patterns seem to be oriented toward diminishing rather than expanding opportunities for exertion. Mechanization of industry, the farm, and the home has been a major factor contributing to a sedentary existence. It has allowed increased production, freedom from hard physical labor, and more leisure time, and has resulted in undeniable conveniences. However, mechanization has been carried to an extreme in some quarters, and society has been conditioned to believe all labor-saving devices are advantageous and that "saving steps" is a goal to aim for in all aspects of life. For instance, the automobile has contributed greatly to an inactive existence, particularly in America, and the American way of life has been geared to driving rather than walking. A neon sign seen when leaving Detroit Metropolitan Airport advised visitors to "automobile city" that: "In this city walking is an insult to American industry." The pleasures and the practicality of both walking and cycling have been ignored. In urban areas, however, it is often faster to travel by bicycle than by car, and when traffic is congested, it is just as fast to walk. Unfortunately under present conditions cyclers and hikers find themselves competing with the automobile, and traveling may often be hazardous. As a final contribution to an inactive existence, modern man has chosen activities during his leisure hours that do not require physical exertion. Radio, television, movies, and spectator sports are the favorite forms of entertainment for many persons.

Man in the modern age has, as described by the British scientists Durnin and Passmore, become "home sedentarius."[30] Such an existence is probably adversely affecting his health. He is obviously not going to return to a laboring existence and a life of drudgery, however he can use his newly acquired leisure time to increase his activity levels. He can become "home sporticus"[31] and perhaps reap the benefits of improved mental and physical health as well as a slim figure. Dancing, games, sports, and tests of strength and physical endurance play a vital role in most cultural patterns and sport is definitely an intrinsic part of American society. Regrettably, however, respect for expertise and the pursuit of inaction has allowed sport to evolve into a phenomenon with few participants and many spectators. Neither the preparation of youth nor the existing sports facilities favor participation by the masses in athletic programs.

For man to become "home sporticus," changes are needed in the attitudes and habits of individuals; but changes are also needed in society and the environment. Community resources in the form of gymnasiums, parks, swimming pools, tennis courts, and safe bicycle paths and footpaths would make an environment conducive to physical activity as a leisure pastime. Hiking and cycling trails, safe from the automobile may encourage individuals to rediscover the beauties of the countryside at a more leisurely pace than is possible from a freeway. Reallocation of funds for these purposes would, however, require a reallignment of priorities in a direction which would be precedent-breaking.

The physical activity habits of adults may be established to a considerable extent in their childhood, just as their food habits often are. If this is the case, it is important that families, schools, and the community encourage habits of exercise in children that will continue through life. School buses, cars, and competitive sports for an elite few have contributed to a population of inactive children. Changes are needed to allow all children as well as adults to reap the benefits and pleasures of regular physical activity and to develop and maintain lifelong patterns of activity.

FOOTNOTES

1. Kraus, H. and Raab, W. *Hypokinetic disease.* Springfield, Ill.: Charles C. Thomas, 1961.
2. Pollack, H. and Consolazio, C. F. Metabolic demands as a factor in weight control. *Journal of the American Medical Association,* 1958, *167,* 216-219.
3. Du Bois, E. F. *Basal metabolism in health and disease.* Philadelphia: Lea and Febiger, 1936.
4. White, R. I., Jr. and Alexander, J. K. Body oxygen consumption and pulmonary ventilation in obese subjects. *Journal of Applied Physiology,* 1965, *20,* 197-201.
5. Present knowledge of calories. *Nutrition Reviews,* 1967, *25,* 257-261.
6. Bogert, J. L., Briggs, G. M., and Calloway, D. H. *Nutrition and physical fitness.* Philadelphia: W. B. Saunders, 1966.
7. Mayer, J. *Overweight: Causes, cost and control.* Englewood Cliffs, N. J.: Prentice-Hall, 1968.
8. *Ibid.*
9. Cunningham, D. A., Montoye, H. J., Metzner, H. L., and Keller, J. B. Active leisure time activities as related to age among males in a total population. *Journal of Gerontology,* 1968, *23,* 551-556.
10. U. S. Department of Agriculture, Economic Research Service. *Food, consumption, prices and expenditures.* (Agricultural Economic Report No. 138) Washington, D.C.: U. S. Government Printing Office, 1968.
11. Du Bois, *op. cit.*
12. Johnson, M. L., Burke, B. S., and Mayer, J. Relative importance of inactivity and overeating in the energy balance of obese high school girls. *American Journal of Clinical Nutrition,* 1956, *4,* 37-44.
13. Stefanik, P. A., Heald, F. P., and Mayer, J. Caloric intake in relation to energy output of nonobese and obese adolescent boys. *American Journal of Clinical Nutrition,* 1959, *7,* 55-62.
14. Bullen, B., Reed, R. B., and Mayer, J. Physical activity of obese and nonobese adolescent girls appraised by motion picture sampling. *American Journal of Clinical Nutrition,* 1964, *14,* 211-223.
15. Chirico, A. M. and Stunkard, A. J. Physical activity and human obesity. *New England Journal of Medicine,* 1960, *263,* 935-940.
16. Dudleston, A. K. and Bennion, M. Effect of diet and/or exercise on obese college women. *Journal of the American Dietetic Association,* 1970, *56,* 126-129.
17. Buskirk, E. R., Thompson, R. H., Lutwak, L., and Whedon, G. D. Energy balance of obese patients during weight reduction: Influence of diet restriction and exercise. *New York Academy of Sciences Annals,* 1963, *110,* 918-939.

18. Exercise for sedentary males. *Nutrition Reviews,* 1970, *28,* 150-151.
19. Mayer, J. Exercise does keep the weight down. *Atlantic Monthly,* 1955, *196,* 66.
20. National Research Council, Food and Nutrition Board. *Recommended Dietary Allowances.* (Publication 1694, 7th rev. ed.) Washington, D.C.: National Academy of Sciences, 1968.
21. Mayer, Exercise does keep the weight down, *op. cit.,* p. 64.
22. Kraus and Raab, *op. cit.* p. iv.
23. Kannel, W. B. The disease of living. *Nutrition Today,* 1971, *6*(3), 2-11.
24. *Ibid.*
25. Skinner, J. S. The cardiovascular system with aging and exercise. In D. Brunner and E. Jokl (Eds.), *Medicine and sport.* Vol. 4. *Physical activity and aging.* Baltimore: University Park Press, 1970.
26. Mann, G. V., Garrett, H. L., Farhi, H., and Billings, F. T. Exercise and heart disease. *American Journal of Medicine,* 1969, *46,* 12-27.
27. Mitrani, Y., Karplus, H., and Brunner, D. Coronary atherosclerosis in cases of traumatic death. In Brunner and Jokl, *Medicine and sport, op. cit.*
28. Kannel, *op. cit.*
29. Cunningham *et al., op. cit.*
30. Durnin, J.V.G.A. and Passmore, R. *Energy, work and leisure.* London: Heinemann Educational Books Ltd., 1967.
31. *Ibid.*

Chapter 7

EXERCISE MANAGEMENT

The benefits of exercise to both general health and the circumference of the waistline have been discussed in the preceding chapter. When considering the sedentary patterns of modern citizens, two general observations can be made. First, there is a lack of awareness of the unusually low levels of physical exertion that are associated with contemporary living conditions. Few people realize, for example, that even military personnel have been observed to spend 88 percent of their day in sedentary activities, with an additional 10 percent spent in light to medium activity and but 2 percent spent in heavy work.[1] Second, even when a need or desire for change in activity levels is felt, it appears to be extremely difficult to modify patterns characterized by inactivity. Dr. Montoye[2] of the University of Michigan observed that physicians have the experience of frequently recommending increased exertion levels but of rarely seeing these recommendations implemented. He commented that it may therefore be easier to establish appropriate patterns of energy expenditure in the first place than to modify patterns already established.

When exercise programs are suggested, the first obstacle encountered is the failure of the overweight person to adequately assess the amount of new exertion which is necessary to produce a useful effect. In the unpublished study cited in Chapter 1, Stuart asked a group of obese women to estimate the amount of exercise required to work off the caloric value of such common foods as doughnuts, ice cream sodas, and potato chips. Comparing their answers to Konishi's[3] figures of 29, 49, and 21 minutes respectively for a 150-pound man walking at the rate of 3.5 miles per hour, they were found to underestimate the true amount of work required by from 200 to 300 percent. This is a reflection of the judgment errors found associated with exertion in a culture which prizes convenience — the expectation of vast return for very moderate change.

The second obstacle encountered is the anticipation of additional fatigue which thereby decreases motivation for exercising. Fatigue arising from daily routine, however, results not so much from activity per se but from the quality of the activity. For example, the modern housewife with small children and the assembly-line worker both experience fatigue, but they are more likely to be suffering from the ill-effects of boredom than the fatigue of physical exertion. Occupations requiring concentrated mental activity may also result in weariness; regrettably, however, the brain does not appear to increase its energy needs when it moves from a relaxed to an active state.[4] The brain has, in fact, been compared to a computer "which use[s] little more electrical current when calculating than when idling."[5] Fatigue resulting from boredom and mental stress must therefore be overcome if efforts to increase exertion levels are to be successful.

The third obstacle which must be overcome is what Dr. D. E. P. Smith[6] of the University of Michigan has termed the "four day phenomenon." This is the four-day period during which dieters, exercisers, and other makers of high-minded resolutions vigorously attack their new way of life, only to find on the fifth day that a dish of ice cream is vitally needed in the middle of the afternoon or that they are just too tired after a day of work to jog around the block. Apparently few of our contemporaries succeed in overcoming the fifth day drop-out point, for the Tecumseh study revealed that the number of consistent exercisers participating in leisure activities requiring a high level of energy expenditure included but 3 percent of the males age 16 to 29 and only 1 percent or less of the 30 to 39 and older age ranges.[7]

The overall picture may not be as bleak as would be implied by the three prepossessing obstacles to exertion. Whether or not the trends can be taken seriously from a health perspective, the soaring sales of exercise gadgets at least reflects an awareness of the need for change toward greater energy expenditure among those with a moderate amount of expendable income. In fact, the number of devices and schemes promising fast health benefits and weight loss is likely to rival the number of fad diets. According to the Family Fitness Council, an association of manufacturers of exercise machines, sales in 1970 ran at almost double those in 1969.[8] It is ironic that a nation which annually devotes billions of dollars to labor-saving machines is now, in addition, spending millions of dollars on labor-making devices. Some undoubtedly serve the purpose for which they are intended, while it is questionable whether others accomplish the dual tasks of weight reduction and physical fitness sought by their owners.

ENERGY EXPENDITURE AND EXERCISE

There are several factors that influence the effect of exertion on caloric expenditure and body fat stores. The involvement and use of large amounts of muscle mass as well as movement of the body weight through distance both have a considerable effect. Thus running that uses most of the larger muscles will expend more energy than pushups, and walking or jogging, more energy than standing and driving a golf ball. In addition, the intensity of exertion affects expenditure considerably, and in a given period of time the more vigorous the exertion the greater will be the caloric expenditure. Therefore a daily 20-minute walk at four miles per hour may use almost twice as many calories as a walk at two miles per hour. Expenditure will naturally vary proportionately with the duration of the activity as well. Furthermore, the conditions of the exertion may also affect energy expenditure. For example, walking on rough ground rather than on smooth, on an incline rather than on the flat or carrying a load rather than not will all increase calorie costs of an activity. Finally,

FIGURE 1
ENERGY EXPENDITURE
WALKING AT DIFFERENT SPEEDS
FOR FIVE SUBJECTS

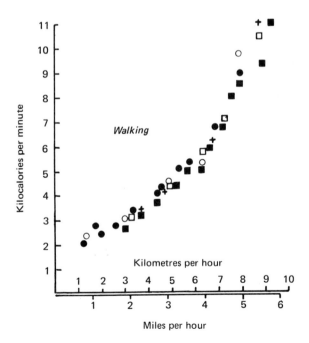

Reproduced with permission from J. V. G. A. Durnin and R. Passmore, *Energy, work and leisure*. London: Heinemann Educational Books Ltd., 1967. P. 41.

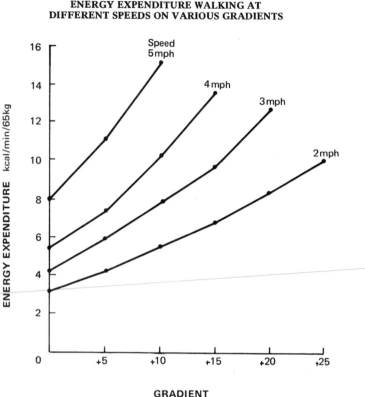

FIGURE 2
ENERGY EXPENDITURE WALKING AT
DIFFERENT SPEEDS ON VARIOUS GRADIENTS

Reproduced with permission from J. V. G. A. Durnin and R. Passmore, *Energy, work and leisure.* London: Heinemann Educational Books Ltd., 1967. P. 44.

individual variability will exert an influence, with the heavy person expending more energy doing a task than his lighter counterpart due to the extra body weight that must be moved; thus the obese individual has an added advantage of greater caloric consumption when exercising. Figures 1 and 2 and Table 1 illustrate the effects of some of these factors on total caloric expenditure.

Measurements of gross energy expenditure have been made on persons involved in a variety of occupations, athletic activities, and other routine tasks (see Appendix F). Some occupations such as mining, lumbering, and farming, especially where mechanization is not available, involve constant heavy labor and may demand caloric expenditures up to or exceeding 10 calories per minute.[9] However, the caloric demands for many occupations such as light industry and household tasks are considerably lower and have decreased with the development of automation. According to Durnin and Passmore, a wide variety of tasks classified as light industry demand energy expenditure rates between 2 and 5 calories per minute for men and 1.5 to 4 calories per minute for women, the rates for women being less due to their lower body weights. They list the energy expenditure of such household activities as dishwashing, cooking, and dusting as between 2 to 2.9 calories per minute for a 120-pound woman.[10] Sedentary occupations demand even lesser caloric expenditure, and Durnin and Passmore list an average value for men of 1.6 calories per minute for office work while sitting and 1.9 calories per minute for work while standing and moving around.[11] Rates measured while lying at rest have been listed as approximately 1.3 calories per minute for a 150-pound man.[12] Table 2 presents an arbitrary example of daily energy expenditure of a 25-year-old man with a body weight of 154 pounds and of a 25-year-old woman with a body weight of 128 pounds. The total expenditures are in accordance with the recommended dietary allowances for calories specified by the Food and Nutrition Board of the National Research Council. It can be seen that routine daily activities use comparatively few calories, that tasks requiring moderate exertion are performed briefly and that regular exercise requiring a high caloric expenditure is not included.

Due to the mechanization of occupational activities and shorter working hours, the type of exercise carried on during leisure time may well make the most significant contribution to daily energy expenditure in modern societies. Figures for leisure activities range from approximately 3

TABLE 1
RELATIONSHIP BETWEEN ENERGY EXPENDITURE
(cal./min.) AND THE SPEED OF WALKING (mph)
AND GROSS BODY WEIGHT (lb.)

Speed, mph	Weight, lb.						
	80	100	120	140	160	180	200
2.0	1.9	2.2	2.6	2.9	3.2	3.5	3.8
2.5	2.3	2.7	3.1	3.5	3.8	4.2	4.5
3.0	2.7	3.1	3.6	4.0	4.4	4.8	5.3
3.5	3.1	3.6	4.2	4.6	5.0	5.4	6.1
4.0	3.5	4.1	4.7	5.2	5.8	6.4	7.0

Reproduced with permission from J. V. G. A. Durnin and R. Passmore, *Energy, work and leisure.* London: Heinemann Educational Books Ltd., 1967. P. 42.

TABLE 2

EXAMPLES OF DAILY ENERGY EXPENDITURES

Activity	Time, hr	Man Rate kcal/min	Man Total	Woman Rate kcal/min	Woman Total
Sleeping and lying (1)	8	1.1	530	1.0	480
Sitting (2)	6	1.5	540	1.1	400
Standing (3)	6	2.5	900	1.5	540
Walking (4)	2	3.0	360	2.5	300
Other (5)	2	4.5	540	3.0	360
Total	24		2880		2100

1   Essentially basal metabolic rate plus some allowance for turning over or getting up or down.
2   Includes normal activity carried on while sitting, e.g., reading, driving an automobile, eating, playing cards, and desk or bench work.
3   Includes normal indoor activities while standing and walking spasmodically in limited areas, e.g., personal toilet, moving from one room to another.
4   Includes purposeful walking, largely outdoors, e.g., home to commuting station to work site, and other comparable activities.
5   Includes spasmodic activities in occasional sports exercises, limited stair climbing, or occupational activities involving light physical work. This category may include weekend swimming, golf, tennis, or picnic using 5 to 20 kcal/min for limited time.

Adapted from National Research Council, Food and Nutrition Board, *Recommended Dietary Allowances.* (Publication 1146, 6th rev. ed.) Washington, D.C.: National Academy of Sciences, 1964.

calories per minute for billiards to 18 calories per minute for cross-country skiing (racing).[13] The expenditure for such activities as volleyball, badminton, and squash average approximately 3.5, 6.3, and greater than 10 calories per minute respectively.[14] Figures for energy expenditures during exercise may however, vary widely depending on the vigor with which the exercise is pursued.

Types of exercise. Exercise, in general, involves work of the skeletal muscles, however different types, intensities, and durations of exercise will have varying effects on the conditioning of the body as well as on caloric expenditure. Passive exercise, where a machine rather than the body muscles are working, results in low levels of caloric expenditure. For example, keeping pace with an electrically driven bicycle involves minimal muscular contraction or work even though the body is moving; expenditure is minimal when compared to a bicycle driven by muscular work. Another type of exercise, often referred to as isometric training, involves muscle contraction but without external gross movement of the body. These exercises tense one set of muscles against another or against an opposing force such as a wall or door frame, the primary purpose being to strengthen and develop individual muscle groups. They may be beneficial in the prevention of muscle atrophy for individuals such as astronauts who are forced to live in confined spaces for prolonged periods of time, but their effectiveness for weight control is probably slight as they neither involve large muscle mass nor gross movement of the body.

Dynamic exercises, on the other hand, involve both muscle contraction plus movement of the body or parts of the body through space, and they will accomplish different physiological results according to their intensity and duration. Some, such as calisthenics, emphasize muscle strength, coordination, and body flexibility. Sports such as bowling, golf, and other less strenuous recreational activities, will have varying effects on caloric expenditure and muscle strength. When carried on continuously they undoubtedly consume energy and use up calories, however when short term and not overly vigorous, their benefit to those seeking weight reduction may be overestimated.

Dynamic exercises of sufficient intensity and duration to demand large amounts of oxygen and increase the work of the heart are often termed aerobic, and when carried out regularly they will train or condition the cardiovascular system. Exercises of very high intensity such as sprints, however, will deplete body hemoglobin and myoglobin oxygen supplies, and under such conditions a portion of the energy comes from anaerobic processes with the eventual result being a physiological demand for termination of the exercise. There is little immediate benefit of such short-term high intensity exercise to the cardiovascular system. Oxygen-demanding exercises of moderate intensity, however, may be carried on for prolonged periods of time without creating an "oxygen debt" and are the recommended form of exercise for conditioning the cardiovascular system. In addition, these exercises have more to offer those seeking weight control or weight maintenance as well. Exercises such as jogging, cycling, swimming, handball, and walking have been recommended for cardiovascular conditioning. The effects of such conditioning may be summarized as follows:

1. An increase in the oxygen-diffusing capacity of the lungs with a correspondingly reduced respiratory rate;

2. An increase in the efficiency of the heart, enabling it to pump more blood with each stroke, thus reducing the number of strokes necessary (bradycardia);

3. An increase in the number and size of the blood vessels carrying blood to the body tissues;

4. An improvement in the tone of the muscles and blood vessels; and

5. An increase in the efficiency of the supply and delivery of oxygen to the working musculature, thus resulting in maximal oxygen consumption and a total increase in aerobic capacity.

In the last decade or so research has developed specific programs for conditioning of the cardiovascular system. A recent paper reviewing patterns of exercise for adults concludes that "training programs are no longer empirical [and] there are several established facts which are of practical value in the planning of exercise patterns of healthy adults."[15] The type of exercise, the intensity, special training methods, the period of time, and specific differences in relation to age, sex, and level of physical condition have all been studied. It has been suggested that a "pharmacopia" of exercise[16] is now available and may be used for individual prescriptions in much the same way medicines are. It is not the purpose of this book to recommend specific conditioning programs but, rather, to suggest ways and means for individuals to increase their caloric expenditure in general. However, excellent books are available outlining in detail such conditioning programs.[17]

EXERCISE MANAGEMENT PLAN

There are, in general, two ways of increasing expenditure that can be incorporated in living patterns. The first attempts to increase expenditure while carrying on the daily occupational and routine activities, e.g., standing rather than sitting to do a job or taking extra steps rather than "saving steps." Such increases in expenditure cannot be measured by any simple method. The second way involves the use of time other than that spent in occupational routine, for example, the participation in some regular form of sport or the use of a bicycle or "shank's mare" for transportation to work. The energy expended during blocks of time devoted to some form of physical exertion can be calculated through the use of the energy expenditure tables, and the effects of such efforts on body weight can thus be monitored.

Exercise as a basic dimension of living. It is necessary to weave increased energy expenditure into the natural fabric of daily living. Although not measurable, such increases will undoubtedly influence caloric expenditure and have some effect on body weight. One should be as conscious of how he uses his body as he is of what he puts into it or how fashionably it is bedecked, but in a labor-saving society this would call for a kind of diurnal heresy. For example, while the telephone company extols the virtues of adding extension telephones to save 70 miles of walking per year, this should be seen by the weight-conscious person as an expensive leisure costing as much as 15 excess pounds of body fat in 10 years.[18] In the same vein, department stores which provide convenient elevators and escalators but poorly lit stairwells cater to the convenience but not the health of their customers, as do the purveyors of golf carts, power (and even riding) lawn mowers, mechanical snow shovels, electric garage doors, carving knives, ice crushers, can openers, toothbrushes, and even parking lots which virtually eliminate walking from shopping tours. To surmount these multifaced forces which would lead to inactivity, one must make a deliberate decision to think before he saves even a single calorie of energy and then act to expend that calorie. This is done by walking upstairs every time it is appropriate instead of waiting for things to accumulate on the bottom step or sending an otherwise quite sufficiently active child up, by sitting instead of lying down, standing instead of sitting, and walking instead of standing every time it is practicable to choose a more energetic option. Finally, while these changes are often more readily arranged in the home, it is also possible to make a number of adjustments in work situations. For example, just using the coat rack and the coffeepot on another floor, using the toilet at the far end of the hall, or parking at the extreme end of the lot can appreciably increase the amount of energy expended over the course of a year. But none of these adjustments will be automatic, some will be the subject of ridicule, and all will require more exertion. To be successful in the face of these odds requires a firm commitment to strongly embracing exertion as a basic thread in the fabric of daily living.

Measurable increases in expenditure. Blocks of exercise taking place during nonoccupational time can be monitored and recorded; moreover, efforts to increase activity during this time will, in general, have the most benefit on total energy expenditure for in modern societies it is recreational rather than occupational activities that, for the most part, demand the greatest physical exertion.

An exercise plan has been developed to allow quick and simple recording of these activities. Various types of exercise have been divided into three general categories—light, moderate, and heavy—and the caloric cost for each type has been estimated (see Table 3). These values are only approximations for they vary with the conditions of the exercise, the size of the individual, and the vigor of the activity. Nevertheless they provide a useful guide for quick calculations of expenditure, and accuracy has been sacrificed for this convenience.

TABLE 3

AVERAGE ENERGY EXPENDITURE
DURING RECREATIONAL ACTIVITIES*

Light Exercise 4 calories/minute	Moderate Exercise 7 calories/minute	Heavy Exercise 10 calories/minute
Dancing (slow step)	Badminton (singles)	Calisthenics (vigorous)
Gardening (light)	Cycling (9.5 mi./hr.)	Climbing stairs (up & down)
Golf	Dancing (fast step)	Cycling (12 mi./hr.)
Table tennis	Gardening (heavy)	Handball, paddleball, squash
Volleyball	Stationary cycling (moderately)	Jogging
Walking (3 mi./hr.)	Swimming (30 yd./min.)	Skipping rope
	Tennis (singles)	Stationary cycling (quickly)
	Walking (4.5 mi./hr.)	Stationary jogging
		Swimming (40 yd./min.)

*Values are for gross energy expenditure.

The exercise plan available with the book should be inserted in the vinyl folder and will allow a daily recording of measurable exercise. Figure 3 illustrates a sample plan which has been recorded. Each box on the plan represents a 5-minute time interval; heavy lines represent 15-minute intervals, and each row represents one hour. An hour's light gardening could account for the one hour of light activity recorded on the plan. A 15-minute brisk walk to and from work could account for the 1/2 hour of moderate activity recorded, and climbing up and down three flights of stairs to a third-floor office three times during the day (each flight of stairs up and down requires approximately 30 seconds) could account for 5 minutes of heavy activity. All of this activity would total 500 calories of energy expenditure.

It is suggested that individuals first gather baseline information regarding their present levels of the activities listed on the exercise plan. Much of the baseline activity will no doubt result from walking, and both walking at a moderate pace and walking briskly have been included. Baseline information may likely include climbing stairs as well. Once baseline information has been derived, it is recommended that individuals then concentrate on increasing this amount by 250 calories each day. Such an increase should result in a weekly weight loss of 1/2 pound and, when coupled with the dietary caloric restriction recommended in Chapter 5, would result in a total weekly loss of 1-1/2 pounds. The daily expenditure over that of the baseline should be recorded on the Eating-Weight-Exercise graph illustrated in Figure 5, Chapter 3 and included at the back of the book. This will permit a comparison of increased exercise, daily caloric intake, and weight loss.

Careful planning and thought is required when contemplating changes in activity levels. Choice of activity will vary with climatic and environmental conditions as well as seasonal changes. Available recreational equipment and facilities will also influence selection of activities. Furthermore, a preference may be had for either a scheduled session of

FIGURE 3
EXERCISE PLAN*

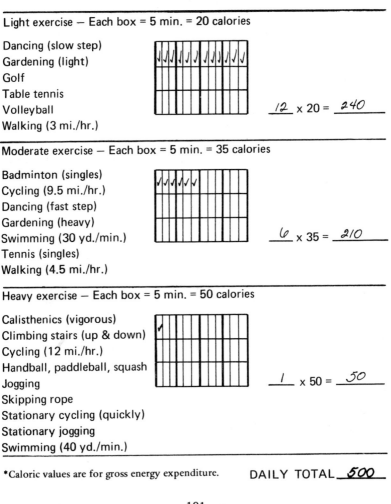

Light exercise — Each box = 5 min. = 20 calories

Dancing (slow step)
Gardening (light)
Golf
Table tennis
Volleyball
Walking (3 mi./hr.)

12 x 20 = *240*

Moderate exercise — Each box = 5 min. = 35 calories

Badminton (singles)
Cycling (9.5 mi./hr.)
Dancing (fast step)
Gardening (heavy)
Swimming (30 yd./min.)
Tennis (singles)
Walking (4.5 mi./hr.)

6 x 35 = *210*

Heavy exercise — Each box = 5 min. = 50 calories

Calisthenics (vigorous)
Climbing stairs (up & down)
Cycling (12 mi./hr.)
Handball, paddleball, squash
Jogging
Skipping rope
Stationary cycling (quickly)
Stationary jogging
Swimming (40 yd./min.)

1 x 50 = *50*

*Caloric values are for gross energy expenditure.   DAILY TOTAL *500* some athletic activity such as tennis or for an activity which is an integrated part of the daily routine such as walking or cycling to work. Whatever the choice, however, it is regular exercise rather than spasmodic activity that is essential.

BEHAVIORAL CONTROL OF EXERCISE

Unfortunately regular exercise is not, at the outset, a richly reinforcing experience for many people and indeed it may actually serve as a "time out" from reinforcement. However the same model of situational control as was found useful in the control of food (see Figure 2, Chapter 3) can be applied to exercise, and it is as essential to manage the situational controls governing the amount and nature of exercise—the antecedents, the response itself, and the consequences—as it is to manage the conditions under which eating occurs.

Some of the antecedents of inactivity must be eliminated. For example, the small refrigerator in the family room which permits the sport spectator to get a can of beer without walking the twenty steps into the kitchen should be removed; the laundry chute which allows the lady of the house to deliver her soiled linens to the basement from the second floor without a step should be taped shut; and it is even helpful to lock the door of the downstairs bathroom so that everyone must climb to the second floor to respond to nature's frequent calls. Also, by parking the car several blocks from the office or shopping area, extra energy must be expended. Other antecedents of inactivity must be suppressed. It is essential, for example, to control fatigue attributable to boredom or lack of sleep as the armchair athlete is unlikely to leave his easy chair if he has the slightest discomfort with which to rationalize inaction. In the same vein, it is wise to establish rules which restrict, for example, the watching of television or the use of the telephone during intervals when exertion should be taking place. Finally, the antecedents of exercise should be strengthened. Thought should be given to the type of activity enjoyed by each person and the basic equipment should be available for each. This may mean the purchase of a tennis racket or bicycle, several people perhaps sharing the cost of more expensive items such as bicycles. It is also helpful to choose to live in areas which have exercise facilities, for example, swimming pools or gyms in apartment buildings, proximity to a "Y" or parks. When these facilities are lacking, it is possible for adults to obtain the resources which are needed, as for example the evening or weekend use of neighborhood school gyms and other facilities. In addition, care should be taken to apprise significant others of exercise intentions so that they can cue exercise in the same appropriate manner as they might cue desirable food selection. Families with small children may need help in arranging for babysitting (e.g., through exchanges with friends) to create the opportunity for exercise, and employers and co-workers might find it expedient to arrange work schedules so as to permit intervals of exercise not normally occurring during the work day.

Probably the single most important antecedent for an effective exercise program is the availability of companionship during the period of exertion. Companionship while exercising can offer dual benefits: Not only will the activity be more pleasurable because of the company, but two or more people can make a commitment to each other to adhere to a decided program. For some individuals the participation in a group activity may be the strongest factor influencing the initiation and continuation of regular periods of exercise. There are several possibilities for this. Community organizations such as the YM-YWCA offer a variety of fitness programs and other forms of recreational activity. There are chapters of the National Jogging Association in many areas; and neighborhoods or co-workers can form *ad hoc* activity groups, utilize school or community facilities, and exercise together. Organizations and clubs might also consider embarking on a program of physical activity as a special project.

As well as making both the social and physical environment conducive to exercise, it is essential that the activity be an enjoyable experience. Exercise should be initiated gradually and increased slowly. Aches and pains resulting from sudden stressful exertion may well end all good intentions to continue exercising. Walking is an excellent form of exercise and the recommended choice for sedentary and/or obese individuals. Companionship, listening to the ball game on a transistor radio, or interesting scenery may all add interest to walking. Once fitness has improved, other activities may be chosen in addition to walking. The frustrations derived from the fiercely competitive attitude that often accompanies organized forms of sport could well be avoided at first, when the goal of regular activity is the personal improvement of fitness and increased caloric expenditure rather than superior levels of proficiency. Thus companionship, commitment, friendly competition, and a preferred choice of activity can make regular exercise enjoyable.

The consequences of exercise are equally important. To reward regular exercise with praise and perhaps more tangible evidence will be an inducement to continue. It will probably also prove influential to keep both the positive consequences of exercising as well as the negative outcomes of inactivity in mind. The method of monitoring activity levels described above permits a simple system for estimating increases in expenditure, cues for increasing expenditure as well as opportunities for social monitoring.

CONCLUSION

The suggestions that have been offered here for increased energy expenditure during both occupational and nonoccupational activities are only a few of the possibilities available. Individuals living in a variety of circumstances and environments will undoubtedly find other ways to increase their own patterns of physical activity. Two precautions are recommended, however, before embarking on a program of increased exertion—first, that the advice of a physician be consulted, and second, that increase be initiated gradually. Sudden exertion can be harmful and spasmodic stressful activity must be avoided. The National Jogging Association offers the following advice:

> Improvement in capacity comes from a gradual increase in the demand placed upon the systems of the body. Patience and prudence must take precedence over haste and heedlessness. Americans are impatient people, addicted to striving for quick results—instantism. But it is safer and more rational, after years of habitual riding in cars and elevators, to walk before jogging and to jog before running.[19]

Once exercise has been gradually accelerated, proficiency gained, and companionship and needed social support provided, it will gradually become an accustomed dimension of the individual's life and, difficult though it may be for comfort lovers to believe, the absence of exercise would actually be sorely missed. Therefore while there are obstacles to the acquisition of a suitable exertion level, once achieved the consequences of exercise perpetuate it.

FOOTNOTES

1. Consolazio, C. F., Johnson, R. E., and Pecora, L. J. *Physiological measurements of metabolic functions in man.* New York: McGraw-Hill, 1963.
2. Montoye, H. J. The role of exercise in preventive medicine. *Journal of Sports Medicine and Physical Fitness,* 1962, 2, 229-232.
3. Konishi, F. Food energy equivalents of various activities. *Journal of the American Dietetic Association,* 1965, 46, 186-188.
4. Durnin, J. V. G. A. and Passmore, R. *Energy, work and leisure.* London: Heinemann Educational Books Ltd., 1967. P. 49.
5. *Ibid.*
6. Smith, D. E. P. Personal communication, January 1968.
7. Cunningham, D. A., Montoye, H. J., Metzner, H. L., and Keller, J. B. Active leisure time activities as related to age among males in a total population. *Journal of Gerontology,* 1968, 23, 551-556.
8. Off the fat of the land. *Newsweek,* April 20, 1970, 86.

9. Astrand, P. and Rodahl, K. *Textbook of work physiology.* New York: McGraw-Hill, 1970.

10. Durnin and Passmore, *op. cit.*

11. *Ibid.*

12. Consolazio, Johnson and Pecora, *op. cit.*

13. Durnin and Passmore, *op. cit.*

14. *Ibid.*

15. Roskamm, H. and Reindell, H. Optimum patterns of exercise for healthy adults. In D. Brunner and E. Jokl (Eds.), *Medicine and sport.* Vol. 4. *Physical activity and aging.* Baltimore: University Park Press, 1970. P. 26.

16. Cooper, K. H. *Aerobics.* New York: M. Evans and Co., 1968.

17. *Ibid.;* Cooper, K. H. *The new aerobics.* New York: M. Evans and Co., 1970; and Bohannon, R. L. and the Consultants of the National Jogging Association. *Guidelines for successful jogging.* Washington D.C.: National Jogging Association, 1970.

18. Mayer, J. *Overweight: Causes, cost and control.* Englewood Cliffs, N. J.: Prentice-Hall, 1968.

19. Bohannon and the Consultants of the National Jogging Association, *op. cit.*

Chapter 8

REQUIEM FOR THE GIRTH OF THE NATION

In 1900, Von Noorden[1] classified all obesities into two major types: "exogenous" obesities attributable to overeating and underexercising, and "endogenous" obesities due to metabolism irregularities. Almost sixty years later Strang[2] broadened the classification to include three types of obesity—an "exogenous" type identical to that of Von Noorden, a "metabolic" type which includes breakdowns in the physiological or psychological regulation of food intake, and an "endogenous" type related to endocrinological dysfunctions of varied sorts. Shortly thereafter Bigsby and Muniz[3] promulgated a fourfold taxonomy of obesity in which each type—"organic or endocrine" obesity, "constitutional or physiological" obesity, "reactive or psychological" obesity, and "other types of obesity"—has from two to twelve subtypes, including, for example, pregnancy and post-partum obesity and lipophobic (fear of becoming fat) conditions as subtypes of reactive or psychological obesity. While Bigsby and Muniz do attempt to differentiate intervention techniques among the varied nosological entities, most of their treatment recommendations revolve around the prudent use of diet instruction, psychological support, and the occasional use of drugs. Viewed against the background of other authors[4] who recommend the use of efforts to rectify the positive energy balance found so often to be associated with obesity, the present plan of decreasing energy intake while increasing energy output has a great range of application. But no program can claim universal applicability, and it is important to specifically cite the limitations of the plan presented in this book.

WHO SHOULD NOT FOLLOW THIS PROGRAM?

The Public Health Service[5] has identified one group of individuals for whom weight loss is contraindicated—those suffering from diverticulitis, gout, and tuberculosis—and another group for whom weight loss is recommended only under very exceptional circumstances—those suffering from Addison's disease, ulcerative colitis, and regional ileitis. For others with atypical, medically relevant conditions such as pregnancy, menopause, or aging, the consultation of a physician is necessary prior to embarking upon a weight-loss program, while for most others the advice of a physician is a desirable antecedent to undertaking such a program. Clearly, then, those who are counseled by their doctors not to start a weight-loss program would be well-advised to follow such a recommendation, and they comprise the first of four groups for which this program is not recommended.

It is unlikely, however, that many people will fall into the group for whom weight loss is imprudent. Instead, most overweight persons can expect encouragement if not frank orders to participate in efforts likely to result in sustainable weight loss. This qualification—"sustainable" weight loss—suggests another group for whom following this program is contraindicated—those seeking short-term weight loss only. It will be recalled that the judgment rendered by the Public Health Service[6] indicated that broad fluctuations in gross body weight may have a more adverse effect upon the level of serum cholesterol and the amount of atherogenic stress than maintenance of a stable, albeit high level of weight. To this risk can be added the probability that those who have failed to sustain earlier weight loss will have a lower probability of sustaining weight lost through subsequent efforts.[7] Therefore those who seek to lose weight for frivolous reasons such as a wish to fit into one's grammar school knickers in order to compete in the geriatrics golf cup championship, to look attractive in a bikini for three weeks of a man-baiting vacation, or to out-slim the bride's parents at a son's wedding can expect their long-range state of health to be impaired through adverse effects upon cholesterol levels and atherogenesis, while at the same time reducing the likelihood of eventual recovery from the problems of overweight.

The association between the motivation for starting weight loss and the likelihood of success can be inferred from observations about weight consciousness in the United States and success in weight-loss treatment in England. Among Americans, consciousness of weight and efforts to diet have been shown to be far more common among women than among men.[8] Women were, in fact, shown to be: (a) more likely than men to view weight as a social liability; (b) more likely than men to reflect excessive weight in concepts of themselves; (c) more likely than men to visibly show the effects of excess weight in their physiques owing to physiological differences; (d) more likely than men to correctly recognize the interaction between overweight and physique; and (e) more vulnerable than men to changes in fashion. Among British Islanders, however, men are more likely to be effective in weight-loss efforts than women.

Summarizing the responses to questionnaires of 1,562 physicians who had treated many thousands of patients for weight reduction, Yudkin stated:

> Men consult their doctors less often about their overweight than do women, but respond better when they do seek advice. The likely reason is that women are more concerned about the aesthetic disadvantages of overweight, but for many of them this is an inadequate incentive to change their diet. Men, on the other hand, are likely to want to reduce their weight only for reasons of health, but, when they do, this incentive is often adequate.[9]

Because seriousness rather than frivolity in initial motivation is surely a factor in the differential outcome of weight loss efforts, two tests should be made to determine whether the probability of sustained weight loss is adequate. First, it is wise to assess the motivation of the would-be weight-loser by asking him to undertake a three-week effort to increase his exertion level. Because exercise often runs counter to America's labor-saving ideal and because exercise is also a means of extending response cost without necessarily also extending the range of immediate reinforcement, exercise management is the aspect of this program which is least likely to be followed. Therefore beginning a manipulation of exercise is an acid test of motivation to participate in the general program, and it has two additional advantages: It is more under the individual's immediate control than are his socially influenced eating patterns, and when undertaken with moderation it is entirely free of undesirable side effects. The moderate and safe exertion-level test of motivation can be as simple as planning a graduated increase in the number of blocks walked by parking the car several blocks from the office or a store, by standing rather than sitting while doing such routine tasks as ironing, and by participating in some form of recreational sport. Adherence to targeted levels of energy expenditure is a good index of the likelihood with which the full plan will be followed.

A second test of the feasibility of success in weight reduction can be obtained from efforts to modify the availability of food in social contexts. Data pertaining to this test can be collected from efforts to:

1. Eliminate three or four types of problematic foods from the house and determine whether other family members promptly replace them;

2. Break down the pairing between eating and social activities such as watching television, attending the movies, or taking a short trip with the family; and

3. Decide upon a direct manipulation of eating responses such as a brief delay, and measure the supportiveness of responses by others, e.g., family members or office mates.

If the observations of the behavior of others who are important prove to be unfavorable following each of these tests, it is wise to undertake a change in the social patterns as a *precondition* to undertaking the recommended program in a comprehensive fashion.

In summary, then, it can be said that four groups of persons should be discouraged from undertaking the proposed plan: those who are advised not to lose weight in the prescribed manner by their physicians, those whose motivation to lose weight is too insubstantial to be likely to sustain the necessary long-term effort, those who fail in efforts to increase their exertion level gradually during a test period, and those for whom little social support will be available for weight-loss efforts. For those not falling within one of these four groups, participation in this program is advisable, however it is essential that each have a clear idea of what to expect.

WHAT SHOULD ONE EXPECT FROM A WEIGHT-REDUCTION PROGRAM?

Repeated observations [10] have revealed that overweight persons undertaking reducing programs associated with diet management can expect to lose more weight initially than over the full course of their efforts. Initial weight loss, lasting for a period of one to three weeks, is attributable essentially to fluid loss. Among women, some of these fluid fluctuations may be associated with the menstrual cycle. For most, however, they are attributable to nutritional chemistry. During these early weeks of dieting, the amount of carbohydrates is reduced. Carbohydrates in the diet have been shown to be associated with the storage of sodium and water in the body. [11] Reduction in carbohydrate intake is therefore reliably associated with loss of fluids which, at 8.2 pounds per gallon, can significantly affect gross body weight. This rapid weight loss is typically followed by a mild rate of weight regain as the body reconstitutes its fluid loss. The essence of weight reduction is, however, fat loss and the temporary regain of weight due to renewed fluid retention is essentially irrelevant to and should not detract from the dieter's enthusiasm for his efforts to lose fat. Furthermore, despite these accelerated periods of weight loss and plateaus associated with weight maintenance, the general pattern of fat removal is highly regular and, according to the findings of Bortz, [12] can be plotted as a linear decelerating function when averaging over plateaus occurring any time there are changes resulting in increased fluid retention—for example, high carbohydrate intake at a holiday meal.

Bearing in mind the rapid initial loss and aperiodic plateaus associated with weight reduction, repeated observations have shown that caloric restriction associated with maintained or moderately increased exertion levels *must produce weight loss overall.* Buskirk and his associates [13] could find no patient who failed to lose weight on diets of less than 1,500 calories; Gordon[14] considers it "thermodynamically impossible" for weight to be maintained on such diets; and the broad experience of nutritionists and physicians generally serves as a basis for a prediction with near-absolute certainty that such diets will be effective. The only pitfalls in the interpretation of weight-loss experience, then, are the possibility of premature discouragement resulting from misinterpretation of the predictable scalloped pattern of expected weight loss and/or disaffiliation resulting from impatience with the one or two pounds per week loss found to be sustainable over time[15] and considered to be prudent.[16] The normal expectation for successful weight-loss programs is, therefore, reduction of gross body weight by an average of from one to two pounds per week over time, with occasional periods of accelerated weight loss interspersed with periods of mild weight gain.

MYTHS TO BE AVOIDED

Once it has been determined that weight loss is prudent for an individual, and once he has adopted a realistic weight-loss objective, he must be careful to avoid several compelling myths as tempting for the reducer as the sirens were for Ulysses. First, he must beware of the *myth that weight loss is easy*. As described in this book, weight loss is a difficult process which requires continuous effort not only by the reducer but by those who must assist him. The effort is found in maintenance of the tactics of situationally controlling the use of food in the environment, in a myriad of decisions which must be made in food selection and preparation, and in the planning and execution of exertion programs. The only means of assuring compliance with the demands of each of these aspects of the program is awareness not only of the prescription but of threats to its actualization, and sustaining this awareness is continuous hard work.

The second fallacy which must be avoided by the successful reducer is the *myth that the rewards of weight loss are immediate*. Weight lost at the prescribed rate of one to two pounds per week leads to very obvious changes in appearance and feelings of vigor only after extended periods of months for the mildly obese and years for the greatly obese. Indeed, exaggerated and premature social reinforcement for appearance changes may in some measure actually encourage the overeater to discontinue or reduce his efforts to lose weight, as found in Stuart's unpublished study of husbands' reactions to weight loss by their spouses. Limited to realistic weight loss, social reinforcement is anything but an immediate consequence of efforts to reduce because meaningful weight loss is slow to occur. Furthermore, the many health benefits associated with weight loss—e.g., lowering of blood pressure, breathlessness, and other symptoms of cardiovascular distress; relief from pain in weight-bearing joints associated with osteoarthritis, intertrigo, and hyperhidrosis; increased glucose tolerance and decreased menstrual disturbances such as dysmenorrhea[17] —may not be associated with weight change until a considerable number of pounds has been lost. Therefore social monitors are well-advised to arrange large amounts of response-contingent reinforcement for efforts made at weight control—e.g., measurement of foods eaten, appropriate food selection, and increases in exertion levels—rather than providing reinforcement only upon the attainment of the ultimate results of these efforts.

The third myth to be avoided is the *myth that the weight-loser can achieve his goals alone.* It is the conclusion of the situational analytic paradigm presented here that while the overweight person must suffer through the physical and social consequences associated with his bulk, he controls neither the etiology nor the maintenance of his obesity. He who would stoically set out to "do it alone" pits himself against all of the forces which have succeeded in creating his problem. Therefore to fail to ask for help is sublime foolishness and to refuse to give it is treachery. On the other hand, to ask for help in harnessing the forces of social influence in the service of weight control is the essence of practicality. It is perhaps this type of reasoning which led the distinguished contributors to the Cornell Conference on Therapy to emphasize that:

> The treatment of obesity is likely to become more successful the less the physician concerns himself with obesity and the more he concerns himself with the obese person and his problems of living. [18]

It follows from the above that artifacts in the treatment of obesity, whether drugs, esoteric devices, or the therapist's unction, may expedite the initiation of weight loss but are unlikely to have any measurable effect over time unless supported by changes in the interaction between the obese individual and those with whom he interacts daily. Therefore it is essential to modify the social environment as a means of achieving lasting weight control, whether this reorganization entails reprogramming the availability or use of food or providing encouraging companions during periods of increased energy expenditure.

The fourth myth to be avoided is the *myth that hunger must be associated with success in weight loss.* In point of fact, it has been repeatedly observed that when weight-losers do experience hunger they frequently deviate from programs of prudent food management and consequently inadvertently overeat. For example, Lewis and Doyle summarized the experiences of 34 successful weight-losers and 22 unsuccessful weight-losers who followed one of three programs. They found that " 'the most successful group' had the highest eating frequency (5.3 times per day),"[19] and it can be concluded from this that the successful group was more likely than their unfortunate counterparts to limit their hunger. When hunger does occur, it is usually followed by intensive eating, a reaction which can only be controlled by the prevention of hunger. Hunger, then, is not a necessary concomitant of weight control but is instead a serious threat to its success.

The fifth myth to be avoided is the *myth that any program is useful for everyone.* Eating patterns develop and are controlled in ways that are highly idiosyncratic. Therefore any effective program must take into account individual preferences for food and unique styles of food management. The food exchange protocol described as part of this program permits individuation of food selections, while the range of techniques available for the situational control of eating is likewise conducive to individualizing the program. For example, one person might minimize the amount that he eats at any given meal by arriving at the table after others have already begun eating, another by choosing to eat only with companions whose eating habits are comparable to those which he seeks for himself, and a third might prepare his meal at home and bring it to work to avoid encountering tempting inappropriate foods in restaurants. Or again, one person might avoid vacations entirely while another might find it expedient to either slightly increase the strength of his diet before a vacation or to plan to increase his exertion level while away from home by staying at a non-centrally located hotel and walking some distance to his amusements or by staying in a room on a high floor and walking up rather than riding the elevator. Adaptation of the program to suit individual preferences in this manner is essential if the program is to prove effective. Furthermore, these adaptations can have the expeditious effect of adding interest to the program, thereby enhancing the likelihood that it will be followed over time. In any case it would be naive to expect that the plan as described here would suit any individual "to a T," and it is therefore essential to make every needed effort to capture in the plan variations which have individual meaning.

The final myth to be avoided is the *myth that weight loss is a short-term effort.* Those programs which can claim effectiveness over time have been identified in Chapter 1 as programs which succeed in reeducating the overeater in techniques necessary for management of his energy balance. The virtue of educational programs is found in their effectiveness in controlling behavior over time, given the gradualness which must typify sustainable weight loss. Therefore any commitment to a weight-loss program must wisely be a commitment for life, for the threats of overeating and underexercising are ubiquitous. When the present program is undertaken it is accordingly strongly recommended that each of the protocols—situational control techniques, the monitoring of eating, and the promulgation of efforts to extend exertion—be systematically reintroduced at intervals not exceeding six months, if only for a seven-day reminder of the details of acceptable practice.

SUMMARY

In summary, it has been stated that the requiem for the girth of the nation can be sung if (a) those for whom weight loss is indicated (b) adopt a realistic goal of losing one to two pounds per week, recognizing that the graph of this loss will display periodic plateaus and short-term weight gain, and (c) follow six recommendations which are the converse of the myths commonly associated with weight loss. These recommendations are:

1. Be prepared to expend effort in losing weight.

2. Be prepared for delayed rather than immediate reinforcement for efforts to lose weight.

3. Draw heavily upon the support of others in the natural—home and work—environment.

4. Avoid hunger through a moderate reduction in diet and increased meal frequency if necessary.

5. Adapt the weight-loss program to individual need.

6. Plan for a continuous change in weight-related behavior, including periodic reinstigation of formal monitoring procedures.

When the general program designed to modify energy balance through the management of the eating environment, food choices, and exertion levels is tempered by the above considerations, success can be expected for a great percentage of those seeking weight loss. Following the recommendations comprising this program, eating behavior can be controlled as readily as any other behavior—e.g., driving on the right side of the road, writing on an even line, or completing a work assignment. The common denominator for all of these behaviors is control of the conditions which set the occasion for the behaviors, arrangement for the needed accelerating consequences to follow the behavior, and direct manipulation of the behaviors in an appropriate manner. When the problem of overeating is approached in this straightforward manner it is as manageable as any other behavior, and this fact should serve as the inspiration for those seeking to bring obesity under control.

FOOTNOTES

1. Von Noorden, C. *Die fettsucht.* Wein: Hoelder, 1900.
2. Strang, J. M. Obesity. In G. G. Duncan (Ed.), *Diseases of metabolism.* Philadelphia: W. B. Saunders, 1959.
3. Bigsby, F. L. and Muniz, C. *Practical management of the obese patient.* New York: Intercontinental Medical Book Corp., 1962.
4. For example, Mayer, J. *Overweight: Causes, cost and control.* Englewood Cliffs, N. J.: Prentice-Hall, 1968; and Gordon, E. S. The present concept of obesity: Etiological factors and treatment. *Medical Times,* 1969, *97,* 142-155.
5. U. S. Public Health Service. *Obesity and health.* Washington, D.C.: U. S. Government Printing Office, undated. P. 51.
6. *Ibid.,* p. 40.
7. Young, C. M., Moore, N. S., Berresford, K., Einset, B. M., and Waldner, B. G. The problem of the obese patient. *Journal of the American Dietetic Association,* 1955, *3,* 1111-1115.
8. Dwyer, J. T., Feldman, J. J., and Mayer, J. The social psychology of dieting. *Journal of Health and Social Behavior,* 1970, *11,* 269-287.
9. Yudkin, J. Doctors' treatment of obesity. *Practitioner,* 1968, *201,* 334.
10. For example, Young *et al., op. cit.*; and Christakis, G. Community programs for weight reduction: Experience of the Bureau of Nutrition, New York City. *Canadian Journal of Public Health,* 1967, *58,* 499-504.
11. Gordon, *op. cit.*
12. Bortz, W. M. Predictability of weight loss. *Journal of the American Medical Association,* 1968, *204,* 99-105.
13. Buskirk, E. R., Thompson, R. H., Lutwak, L., and Whedon, G. D. Energy balance of obese patients during weight reduction: Influence of diet restriction and exercise. *New York Academy of Sciences Annals,* 1963, *110,* 918-939.
14. Gordon, *op. cit.*
15. McLaren, B. A. Nutritional control of overweight. *Canadian Journal of Public Health,* 1967, *58,* 483-485.
16. Wang, R. I. H. and Sandoval, R. Current status of therapy in management of obesity. *Wisconsin Medical Journal,* 1969, *68,* 219-220.
17. Gelvin, E. P. and McGavack, T. H. *Obesity: Its cause, classification and cure.* New York: Hoeber-Harper, 1957. Pp. 130-132.
18. Cornell Conferences on Therapy. The management of obesity. *New York State Journal of Medicine,* 1958, *58,* 82.
19. Lewis, K. J. and Doyle, M. D. Nutrient intake and weight response of women on weight-control diets. *Journal of the American Dietetic Association,* 1970, *56,* 124.

APPENDIX A

MEDIAN AND QUARTILE WEIGHT[1] FOR MEN AND WOMEN, BY AGE AND HEIGHT: UNITED STATES, 1960-62[2]

Ht.	Total, 18-79 years			18-24 years			25-34 years			35-44 years		
	P_{25}	P_{50}	P_{75}	P_{25}	P_{50}	P_{75}	P_{25}	P_{50}	P_{75}	P_{25}	P_{50}	P_{75}
Men					Weight in pounds							
62"	128	144	164	122	132	175	131	141	152	141	146	152
63"	134	151	163	127	138	162	130	151	158	132	158	178
64"	136	155	167	121	128	156	129	147	163	137	158	167
65"	139	157	177	131	139	159	129	156	174	151	165	183
66"	144	160	177	141	153	170	144	160	174	151	162	180
67"	146	162	180	138	151	168	147	164	187	150	163	178
68"	149	166	185	144	153	168	146	159	182	154	168	184
69"	153	172	187	145	161	184	156	174	188	156	175	189
70"	159	176	195	148	163	177	163	178	196	164	179	195
71"	166	182	201	152	163	177	163	180	200	175	186	204
72"	162	179	198	153	166	183	169	188	208	165	182	197
73"	177	188	208	171	184	195	178	188	206	184	191	202
74"	166	188	209	164	174	207	164	183	201	203	211	215
Women												
57"	119	130	149	[3]98	[3]116	[3]133	[3]90	[3]112	[3]133	115	125	132
58"	109	129	147	101	107	155	103	110	118	107	118	132
59"	114	130	149	98	112	142	104	118	131	113	128	157
60"	117	133	150	106	117	131	112	123	138	116	132	156
61"	119	137	156	110	121	136	112	120	143	118	130	151
62"	119	136	158	113	125	143	115	127	145	119	135	159
63"	123	137	158	113	122	132	115	128	145	125	138	160
64"	124	138	159	116	126	136	122	133	152	126	140	158
65"	126	139	157	118	132	143	124	134	157	121	137	154
66'	128	140	158	124	137	148	125	136	146	133	142	160
67"	134	152	177	123	134	148	131	147	171	132	150	178
68"	128	147	165	120	129	145	118	147	163	131	148	168

[1]Median—P_{50}, the percentile below which 50 percent of the population fall. Quartiles—P_{25} and P_{75}, the 25th and 75th percentile below which 25 and 75 percent of the population fall.

[2]Height without shoes; weight partially clothed—clothing weight estimated as averaging 2 pounds.

Ht.	45-54 years			55-64 years			65-74 years			75-79 years		
	P_{25}	P_{50}	P_{75}	P_{25}	P_{50}	P_{75}	P_{25}	P_{50}	P_{75}	P_{25}	P_{50}	P_{75}

Men   Weight in pounds

Ht.	P_{25}	P_{50}	P_{75}	P_{25}	P_{50}	P_{75}	P_{25}	P_{50}	P_{75}	P_{25}	P_{50}	P_{75}
62"	131	140	149	115	134	183	155	164	169	122	161	166
63"	137	150	164	140	153	162	140	154	167	126	139	146
64"	150	159	176	141	158	170	142	162	167	129	136	144
65"	143	161	182	137	150	168	137	155	181	140	160	165
66"	148	162	180	145	166	181	137	159	174	138	151	159
67"	151	165	188	148	168	187	141	159	172	145	183	193
68"	153	174	189	153	173	182	147	160	181	163	191	202
69"	153	173	190	161	173	185	141	149	186	138	148	174
70"	164	182	200	151	162	200	166	177	188	[3]156	[3]174	[3]191
71"	174	187	208	166	177	194	157	183	204	[3]162	[3]179	[3]196
72"	170	184	197	162	172	203	[3]159	[3]178	[3]198	[3]167	[3]184	[3]201
73"	167	178	215	205	214	224	[3]162	[3]182	[3]201	[3]172	[3]189	[3]206
74"	150	187	253	[3]171	[3]191	[3]211	[3]166	[3]185	[3]204	[3]177	[3]194	[3]212

Women

Ht.	P_{25}	P_{50}	P_{75}	P_{25}	P_{50}	P_{75}	P_{25}	P_{50}	P_{75}	P_{25}	P_{50}	P_{75}
57"	115	138	166	122	126	130	125	144	150	120	125	130
58"	103	116	130	126	136	148	119	141	159	120	135	163
59"	119	131	148	123	137	149	121	142	160	118	130	146
60"	119	133	150	133	149	165	130	139	154	118	152	162
61"	130	145	166	131	143	162	131	145	162	115	149	183
62"	121	139	159	135	152	178	130	153	172	114	135	154
63"	126	141	160	135	149	180	132	144	163	122	146	156
64"	133	150	176	133	149	176	136	157	174	131	155	191
65"	136	149	177	143	149	184	128	146	157	[3]133	[3]153	[3]173
66"	141	156	175	125	138	165	122	164	182	[3]137	[3]157	[3]176
67"	149	159	179	156	179	186	[3]147	[3]166	[3]185	[3]140	[3]160	[3]180
68"	145	155	170	129	157	180	[3]150	[3]170	[3]189	[3]144	[3]164	[3]183

[3]Estimated values obtained from the linear regression equations.

From U. S. Public Health Service, *Weight, height, and selected body dimensions of adults: United States, 1960-1962.* Washington, D.C.: U. S. Government Printing Office, 1965. Pp. 12-13.

APPENDIX B

FOOD AND NUTRITION BOARD, NATIONAL ACADEMY OF SCIENCES—NATIONAL RESEARCH COUNCIL RECOMMENDED DAILY DIETARY ALLOWANCES,° REVISED 1968

Designed for the maintenance of good nutrition of practically all healthy people in the U.S.A.

	AGE[b]	WEIGHT		HEIGHT			Protein	FAT-SOLUBLE VITAMINS		
								Vitamin A Activity (IU)	Vitamin D (IU)	Vitamin E Activity (IU)
	years	kg	lbs.	cm	in.	kcal	(gm)			
Infants	0–1/6	4	9	55	22	kg X 120	kg X 2.2[e]	1,500	400	5
	1/6–1/2	7	15	63	25	kg X 110	kg X 2.0[e]	1,500	400	5
	1/2–1	9	20	72	28	kg X 100	kg X 1.8[e]	1,500	400	5
Children	1–2	12	26	81	32	1,100	25	2,000	400	10
	2–3	14	31	91	36	1,250	25	2,000	400	10
	3–4	16	35	100	39	1,400	30	2,500	400	10
	4–6	19	42	110	43	1,600	30	2,500	400	10
	6–8	23	51	121	48	2,000	35	3,500	400	15
	8–10	28	62	131	52	2,200	40	3,500	400	15
Males	10–12	35	77	140	55	2,500	45	4,500	400	20
	12–14	43	95	151	59	2,700	50	5,000	400	20
	14–18	59	130	170	67	3,000	60	5,000	400	25
	18–22	67	147	175	69	2,800	60	5,000	400	30
	22–35	70	154	175	69	2,800	65	5,000	—	30
	35–55	70	154	173	68	2,600	65	5,000	—	30
	55–75+	70	154	171	67	2,400	65	5,000	—	30
Females	10–12	35	77	142	56	2,250	50	4,500	400	20
	12–14	44	97	154	61	2,300	50	5,000	400	20
	14–16	52	114	157	62	2,400	55	5,000	400	25
	16–18	54	119	160	63	2,300	55	5,000	400	25
	18–22	58	128	163	64	2,000	55	5,000	400	25
	22–35	58	128	163	64	2,000	55	5,000	—	25
	35–55	58	128	160	63	1,850	55	5,000	—	25
	55–75+	58	128	157	62	1,700	55	5,000	—	25
Pregnancy						+200	65	6,000	400	30
Lactation						+1,000	75	8,000	400	30

° The allowance levels are intended to cover individual variations among most normal persons as they live in the United States under usual environmental stresses. The recommended allowances can be attained with a variety of common foods, providing other nutrients for which human requirements have been less well defined.

[b] Entries on lines for age range 22-35 years represent the reference man and woman at age 22. All other entries represent allowances for the midpoint of the specified age range.

Ascorbic Acid (mg)	Folacin (mg)[c]	Niacin (mg equiv)[d]	Riboflavin (mg)	Thiamin (mg)	Vitamin B6 (mg)	Vitamin B12 (µg)	Calcium (g)	Phosphorus (g)	Iodine (µg)	Iron (mg)	Magnesium (mg)
35	0.05	5	0.4	0.2	0.2	1.0	0.4	0.2	25	6	40
35	0.05	7	0.5	0.4	0.3	1.5	0.5	0.4	40	10	60
35	0.1	8	0.6	0.5	0.4	2.0	0.6	0.5	45	15	70
40	0.1	8	0.6	0.6	0.5	2.0	0.7	0.7	55	15	100
40	0.2	8	0.7	0.6	0.6	2.5	0.8	0.8	60	15	150
40	0.2	9	0.8	0.7	0.7	3	0.8	0.8	70	10	200
40	0.2	11	0.9	0.8	0.9	4	0.8	0.8	80	10	200
40	0.2	13	1.1	1.0	1.0	4	0.9	0.9	100	10	250
40	0.3	15	1.2	1.1	1.2	5	1.0	1.0	110	10	250
40	0.4	17	1.3	1.3	1.4	5	1.2	1.2	125	10	300
45	0.4	18	1.4	1.4	1.6	5	1.4	1.4	135	18	350
55	0.4	20	1.5	1.5	1.8	5	1.4	1.4	150	18	400
60	0.4	18	1.6	1.4	2.0	5	0.8	0.8	140	10	400
60	0.4	18	1.7	1.4	2.0	5	0.8	0.8	140	10	350
60	0.4	17	1.7	1.3	2.0	5	0.8	0.8	125	10	350
60	0.4	14	1.7	1.2	2.0	6	0.8	0.8	110	10	350
40	0.4	15	1.3	1.1	1.4	5	1.2	1.2	110	18	300
45	0.4	15	1.4	1.2	1.6	5	1.3	1.3	115	18	350
50	0.4	16	1.4	1.2	1.8	5	1.3	1.3	120	18	350
50	0.4	15	1.5	1.2	2.0	5	1.3	1.3	115	18	350
55	0.4	13	1.5	1.0	2.0	5	0.8	0.8	100	18	350
55	0.4	13	1.5	1.0	2.0	5	0.8	0.8	100	18	300
55	0.4	13	1.5	1.0	2.0	5	0.8	0.8	90	18	300
55	0.4	13	1.5	1.0	2.0	6	0.8	0.8	80	10	300
60	0.8	15	1.8	+0.1	2.5	8	+0.4	+0.4	125	18	450
60	0.5	20	2.0	+0.5	2.5	6	+0.5	+0.5	150	18	450

[c] The folacin allowances refer to dietary sources as determined by *Lactobacillus casei* assay. Pure forms of folacin may be effective in doses less than ¼ of the RDA.

[d] Niacin equivalents include dietary sources of the vitamin itself plus 1 mg equivalent for each 60 mg of dietary tryptophan.

[e] Assumes protein equivalent to human milk. For proteins not 100 percent utilized factors should be increased proportionately.

APPENDIX C

FOOD EXCHANGE LISTS

All foods within each exchange list, in the amounts specified, are approximately equal in caloric content. It is essential that foods be weighed or measured until portions can be estimated accurately.

CALORIE-FREE FOODS

The following foods, seasonings, and beverages either have negligible calories or no calories at all. They may be used freely in reasonable amounts and do not have to be recorded on the daily food plan.

All raw vegetables from the **vegetable** exchange list

Bouillon

Broths, clear (no fat)

Coffee

Cranberries (unsweetened)

Garlic

Gelatin (unflavored)

Herbs

Horseradish

Lemon juice

Lime juice

Mustard

Onion flakes

Pickles (dill, unsweetened)

Pickles (sour)

Rennet tablets

Rhubarb (unsweetened)

Saccharin

Soy sauce

Spices

Tea

Vinegar

MEAT EXCHANGE LIST

Each meat exchange supplies approximately 75 calories of energy. The lean meats will average somewhat less than this amount and the fat meats somewhat more. An average serving portion of *cooked* meat weighs approximately 3 ounces, which would be *3* meat exchanges. At least 2 serving portions of meat or meat products (6 exchanges) should be eaten daily.

List 1. The following are *lean* meats and *low-fat* cheeses, and increased use of these is encouraged:

Exchange	Amount to Use for 1 Exchange
Meat and poultry	
Chicken, game meats, liver and other organ meats, pheasant, rabbit, turkey, veal	1 ounce
Fish	
Bass, cod, flounder, haddock, halibut, lobster, salmon, trout, etc.	1 ounce
Crab, lobster, salmon, tuna	¼ cup (loosely packed)
Clams, oysters, scallops, shrimp	3-5 medium
Cheese	
Cottage cheese	1/3 cup
Skimmed or partially skimmed milk	1 1-inch cube or 1 ounce

List 2. The following meat exchanges contain *more fat;* these should be used more sparingly.

Meat and poultry	
Beef, duck, goose, ham, lamb, pork	1 ounce
Eggs	1 egg
Cheese	
American (processed), cheddar, Edam, Swiss, etc.	1 slice (4 x 4 x 1/8 inches) or 1 1-inch cube or 1 ounce
Peanut butter	1 tablespoon
Cold cuts - bologna, salami, etc.	1 slice (4½ x 4½ x 1/8 inches)
Frankfurters (8-9 per lb.)	1 small
Sausage	1 small link

CEREAL EXCHANGE LIST

Each cereal exchange supplies approximately 70 calories of energy. Soups and high-carbohydrate vegetables have been included on the cereal exchange list. At least three servings of whole grain or enriched breads or cereals should be eaten daily.

Exchange	Amount to Use for 1 Exchange
Breads and rolls	
Bagel	½
Bread dressing or stuffing	2 tablespoons
Hamburger, hot dog bun (large)	½ bun
Matzos	1 6-inch diameter
White, whole-wheat, rye	1 slice
Quick breads	
Biscuit, roll, muffin	1 2-inch diameter
Corn bread	1 piece 1½-inch cube
Doughnut, plain	1 small
English muffin	½
Pancake	1 4-inch diameter cake
Waffle	1 4-inch diameter waffle
Crackers	
Graham	2 crackers, 2½-inches square
Oyster	½ cup
Round	5 crackers, 2-inches diameter
Rye	2 double crackers
Saltines	5 crackers, 2-inches square
Soda	3 crackers, 2½-inches square
Cereals	
Cooked: grits, oats, rice, wheat	½ cup
Ready-to-eat: flake and puff types	¾ cup
Pastas (cooked, noodles only)	
Egg noodles, macaroni, spaghetti	½ cup
Flour	2½ tablespoons
Vegetables and soups	
Baked beans in sauce (no pork)	¼ cup
Corn	1 small ear or ½ cup kernels
Dried beans, lentils, peas (cooked)	½ cup
Parsnips	½ cup
Popcorn (no butter)	1 cup
Potatoes	1 small or ½ cup mashed
Potatoes, sweet or yams	¼ cup
Tomato sauce or catsup	¼ cup
Soup, meat or vegetable	1 serving (3 per can)
Soup, cream, pea, or bean	½ serving (3 per can)

MILK EXCHANGE LIST

Each milk exchange supplies approximately 85 calories of energy. Skimmed or partially skimmed milk should be used. Two cups of milk or its equivalent should be drunk daily.

Exchange	Amount to Use for 1 Exchange
Buttermilk (skimmed)	1 cup (8 ounces)
Cottage cheese (creamed)	1/3 cup
Cottage cheese (plain)	½ cup
Evaporated milk	¼ cup
Evaporated milk (skimmed)	½ cup
Ice milk	1/3 cup
Nonfat dried milk powder	¼ cup
Partially skimmed milk	¾ cup
Skimmed milk	1 cup
Yogurt, plain (made from partially skimmed milk)	¾ cup
Yogurt, plain (made from skimmed milk)	1 cup
Yogurt, fruit and flavored	½ cup

VEGETABLE EXCHANGE LIST

Three vegetable exchanges (two from the first list and one from the second) supply approximately 50 calories. The vegetables in bold type are especially rich sources of vitamins. At least two servings of vegetables should be eaten daily, including one vitamin-rich vegetable.

List 1. The following vegetables provide negligible calories. In raw form they may be eaten as desired in reasonable amounts and do not need to be recorded on the daily food plan. When cooked, limit serving portions to ½ to 1 cup and record as one vegetable exchange.

Asparagus	**Collards**
Bamboo shoots	**Dandelion greens**
Broccoli	**Kale**
Brussels sprouts	**Mustard greens**
Cabbage	**Spinach**
Cauliflower	**Turnip greens**
Celery	Kohlrabi
Cucumber	Lettuce
Eggplant	Mushrooms
Endive	Okra
Green beans, young	**Peppers**
Green onions	Radishes
Greens	Sauerkraut
Beet greens	Summer squash
Chard	**Watercress**

List 2. The following vegetables contain more carbohydrates and therefore provide more calories. When cooked, average one serving of these vegetables daily, but limit serving portions to ½ cup and count as one vegetable exchange. When used in the raw form, it is not necessary to record these as a vegetable exchange on the daily food plan, but use these raw vegetables less frequently than those from List 1.

Artichokes	Pea pods
Beets	**Pumpkin**
Carrots	Rutabagas
Onions	Turnips
Peas	**Winter squash**

FRUIT EXCHANGE LIST

Each fruit exchange provides approximately 40 calories of energy. Fruits may be fresh, dried, cooked, canned, or frozen as long as *no sugar* is added. Those in bold type are especially rich in vitamin C. Two exchanges of fruit should be eaten daily, with at least one being a vitamin C-rich fruit.

Exchange	Amount to Use for 1 Exchange
Apple	1 small or ½ medium
Apple juice	½ cup
Applesauce	½ cup
Apricots	2
Apricots, dried	4 halves
Banana	½ small
Blackberries	1 cup
Blueberries	1 cup
Cantaloupe	¼ small
Cherries	12
Figs, fresh	2
Grapes	12
Grape juice	¼ cup
Grapefruit	½ small
Grapefruit juice	½ cup
Guava	1
Honeydew melon	1/8
Mango	½ small
Orange	1 small
Orange juice	½ cup
Papaya	½ small
Peach	1
Pear	1 small
Pineapple	½ cup
Pineapple juice	½ cup
Plums	2
Raisins	2 tablespoons
Raspberries	1 cup
Strawberries	1 cup
Tomato	1 large
Tomato juice	1 cup
Watermelon	1 cup

MISCELLANEOUS FOODS EXCHANGE LIST

These foods and beverages provide concentrated sources of calories. Those in bold type supply only calories and are called "empty calorie foods." They should be used sparingly.

List 1 (Fats). Each of these provides approximately 40 calories per exchange. Those in italics are good sources of polyunsaturated fatty acids.

Exchange	Amount to Use for 1 Exchange
Avocado	1/8 4-inch diameter
Bacon, crisp	1 slice
Butter or *margarine*	1 teaspoon
Cream, light	2 tablespoons
Cream, heavy or sour	1 tablespoon
Cream cheese	1 tablespoon
French dressing	1 tablespoon
Mayonnaise	1 teaspoon
Nuts	6 small
Oil or cooking fat	1 teaspoon
Olives	5 small

List 2 (Sweets). The following sweets provide approximately 40 calories per exchange.

Exchange	Amount to Use for 1 Exchange
Cocoa (sweetened)	1 level tablespoon or 1 heaping teaspoon
Hard candy (small) or caramel	1
Sugar, syrup, honey, jam, jelly	1 level tablespoon or 1 heaping teaspoon

List 3 (Desserts and beverages). These foods, in the amounts specified, supply approximately 80 calories and must be counted as *2* miscellaneous food exchanges.

Exchange	Amount to Use for 2 Exchanges
Desserts	
Cake: sponge, angel food, made with enriched flour	1 piece, 2 x 2 x 1 inches
Jello	1 serving (5 per package)
Sherbet	1/3 cup
Any dessert, if 1 serving portion is no more than 80 calories	1 serving
Beverages	
Beer	6 ounces
Carbonated beverages	6 ounces
Gin, rum, whiskey †	1 ounce
Liqueur (creme de menthe, etc.)	1 ounce
Wine (red, sweet)	2 ounces
Wine (light, dry)	3 ounces

† Note that one jigger is 1½ ounces and would be counted as *3* miscellaneous food exchanges.

APPENDIX D

EQUIVALENTS BY VOLUME

(All measurements level)

1 quart	=	4 cups
1 cup	=	8 fluid ounces
	=	½ pint
	=	16 tablespoons
2 tablespoons	=	1 fluid ounce
1 tablespoon	=	3 teaspoons
1 pound regular butter or margarine	=	4 sticks
1 pound whipped butter or margarine	=	2 cups
	=	6 sticks
	=	2 8-ounce containers
	=	3 cups

APPENDIX E

NUTRITIVE VALUES OF THE EDIBLE PART OF FOODS

Food	Measure	Food Energy calories*	Protein grams	Fat grams	Carbohydrate grams
MILK, CHEESE, CREAM, IMITATION CREAM; RELATED PRODUCTS					
Milk:					
Fluid:					
Whole, 3.5% fat	1 cup	160	9	9	12
Nonfat (skim)	1 cup	90	9	Trace	12
Canned, concentrated, undiluted:					
Evaporated, unsweetened	1 cup	345	18	20	24
Condensed, sweetened	1 cup	980	25	27	166
Dry, nonfat instant:					
Low-density (1-1/3 cups needed for reconstitution to 1 qt.)	1 cup	245	24	Trace	35
High-density (7/8 cup needed for reconstitution to 1 qt.)	1 cup	375	37	1	54
Buttermilk (fluid, cultured, made from skim milk)	1 cup	90	9	Trace	12
Cheese:					
Natural:					
Blue or Roquefort type	1 oz.	105	6	9	1
Cheddar	1 oz.	115	7	9	1
Cottage, large or small curd, creamed, curd pressed down	1 cup	260	33	10	7
Cream	1 oz.	105	2	11	18
Parmesan, grated	1 tbsp.	25	2	2	Trace
Swiss	1 oz.	105	8	8	1
Pasteurized processed cheese:					
American	1 oz.	105	7	9	1
Swiss	1 oz.	100	8	8	1

Food	Measure	Food Energy calories*	Protein grams	Fat grams	Carbohydrate grams
Pasteurized processed cheese food, American	1 tbsp.	45	3	3	1
Pasteurized process cheese spread, American	1 oz.	80	5	6	2
Cream:					
Half-and-half (cream and milk)	1 tbsp.	20	1	2	1
Light, coffee or table	1 tbsp.	30	1	3	1
Sour	1 tbsp.	25	Trace	2	1
Whipped topping (pressurized)	1 tbsp.	10	Trace	1	Trace
Imitation cream products (made with vegetable fat):					
Creamers:					
Powdered	1 tbsp.	10	Trace	1	1
Liquid (frozen)	1 tbsp.	20	Trace	2	2
Whipped topping (pressurized, frozen or powdered, made with whole milk)	1 tbsp.	10	Trace	1	1
Milk beverages:					
Cocoa, homemade	1 cup	245	10	12	27
Malted milk	1 cup	245	11	10	28
Milk desserts:					
Custard, baked	1 cup	305	14	15	29
Ice cream:					
Regular (10% fat)	1 cup	255	6	14	28
Rich (16% fat)	1 cup	330	4	24	27
Ice milk:					
Hardened	1 cup	200	6	7	29
Soft-serve	1 cup	265	8	9	39
Yogurt (made from partially skimmed milk)	1 cup	125	8	4	13

EGGS

Eggs, large, 24 oz. per dozen:
Raw or cooked in shell or with nothing added:

Whole, without shell	1 egg	80	6	6	Trace
White of egg	1 white	20	4	Trace	Trace
Yolk of egg	1 yolk	60	2	5	Trace
Scrambled with milk and fat	1 egg	110	7	8	1

MEAT, POULTRY, FISH, SHELLFISH; RELATED PRODUCTS

Bacon (20 slices per lb.) broiled or fried, crisp	2 slices	90	5	8	1
Beef, cooked:					
Cuts braised, simmered, or pot-roasted:					
Lean and fat	3 oz.	245	23	16	0
Lean only	3 oz.	170	26	6	0
Hamburger (ground beef), broiled:					
Lean	3 oz.	185	23	10	0
Regular	3 oz.	245	21	17	0
Roast, oven-cooked, no liquid added:					
Relatively fat, such as rib:					
Lean and fat	3 oz.	375	17	34	0
Lean only	3 oz.	210	23	11	0
Relatively lean, such as heel of round:					
Lean and fat	3 oz.	165	25	7	0
Lean only	3 oz.	140	26	3	0
Steak, broiled:					
Relatively fat, such as sirloin:					
Lean and fat	3 oz.	330	20	27	0
Lean only	3 oz.	175	27	6	0

Food	Measure	Food Energy calories*	Protein grams	Fat grams	Carbohydrate grams
Relatively lean, such as round:					
Lean and fat	3 oz.	220	24	13	0
Lean only	3 oz.	165	26	5	0
Beef, canned:					
Corned beef	3 oz.	185	22	10	0
Corned beef hash	3 oz.	155	7	10	9
Beef, dried or chipped	2 oz.	115	19	4	0
Chicken, cooked:					
Flesh only, broiled	3 oz.	115	20	3	0
Breast, fried, ½ breast (with bone add 0.6 oz.)	2.7 oz.	155	25	5	1
Drumstick, fried (with bone add 0.8 oz.)	1.3 oz.	90	12	4	Trace
Chicken, canned, boneless	3 oz.	170	18	10	0
Chili con carne, canned:					
With beans	1 cup	335	19	15	30
Without beans	1 cup	510	26	38	15
Heart, beef, lean, braised	3 oz.	160	27	5	1
Lamb, cooked:					
Chop, thick, with bone, broiled, 4.8 oz.	1 chop	400	25	33	0
Lean and fat	3 oz.	300	19	25	0
Lean only	3 oz.	160	24	7	0
Leg, roasted:					
Lean and fat	3 oz.	235	22	16	0
Lean only	3 oz.	155	23	6	0
Shoulder, roasted:					

222

	Amount	Calories			
Lean and fat	3 oz.	285	18	23	0
Lean only	3 oz.	170	23	8	0
Liver, beef, fried	2 oz.	130	15	6	3
Pork, cured, cooked:					
Ham, light cure, lean and fat, roasted	3 oz.	245	18	19	0
Luncheon meat:					
Boiled ham, sliced	2 oz.	135	11	10	0
Canned, spiced or unspiced	2 oz.	165	8	14	1
Pork, fresh, cooked:					
Chop, thick with bone (3.5 oz.)	1 chop	260	16	21	0
Lean and fat	3 oz.	340	21	27	0
Lean only	3 oz.	230	26	12	0
Roast, oven-cooked, no liquid added:					
Lean and fat	3 oz.	310	21	24	0
Lean only	3 oz.	220	25	13	0
Cuts, simmered:					
Lean and fat	3 oz.	320	20	26	0
Lean only	3 oz.	185	25	8	0
Sausage:					
Bologna, slice, 3-inch diam. by 1/8 inch	2 slices	80	3	7	Trace
Frankfurter, heated (8 per lb. purchased pkg.)	1 frank	170	7	15	1
Pork links, cooked (16 links per lb. raw)	2 links	125	5	11	Trace
Salami, dry type	1 oz.	130	7	11	Trace
Salami, cooked	1 oz.	90	5	7	Trace
Veal, medium fat, cooked, bone removed:					
Cutlet	3 oz.	185	23	9	Trace
Roast	3 oz.	230	23	14	0
Fish and shellfish:					
Clams, raw, meat only	3 oz.	65	11	1	2
Crabmeat, canned	3 oz.	85	15	2	1

Food	Measure	Food Energy calories*	Protein grams	Fat grams	Carbohydrate grams
Fish sticks, breaded, cooked, frozen; stick 3¾ by 1 by ½ inch	10 sticks or 8 oz. pkg.	400	38	20	15
Haddock, breaded, fried	3 oz.	140	17	5	5
Ocean perch, breaded, fried	3 oz.	195	16	11	6
Oysters, raw, meat only (13-19 med. selects)	1 cup	160	20	4	8
Salmon, pink, canned	3 oz.	120	17	5	0
Sardines, Atlantic, canned in oil, drained solids	3 oz.	175	20	9	0
Shrimp, canned, meat	3 oz.	100	21	1	1
Tuna, canned in oil, drained solids	3 oz.	170	24	7	0

MATURE DRY BEANS AND PEAS, NUTS, PEANUTS; RELATED PRODUCTS

Food	Measure	Food Energy calories*	Protein grams	Fat grams	Carbohydrate grams
Almonds, shelled, whole kernels	1 cup	850	26	77	28
Beans, dry:					
Cooked, drained:					
Great Northern	1 cup	210	14	1	38
Navy (pea)	1 cup	225	15	1	40
Canned, solids and liquid:					
White with pork and tomato sauce	1 cup	310	16	7	49
Red kidney	1 cup	230	15	1	42
Peanuts, roasted, salted, halves	1 cup	840	37	72	27
Peanut butter	1 tbsp.	95	4	8	3
Peas, split, dry, cooked	1 cup	290	20	1	52

VEGETABLES AND VEGETABLE PRODUCTS

Asparagus, green, pieces, cooked, drained	1 cup	30	3	Trace	5
Beans:					
Lima, immature seeds, cooked, drained	1 cup	190	13	1	34
Snap:					
Green, cooked, drained	1 cup	30	2	Trace	7
Yellow or wax, cooked, drained	1 cup	30	2	Trace	6
Sprouted mung beans, cooked, drained	1 cup	35	4	Trace	7
Beets, diced or sliced, cooked, drained	1 cup	55	2	Trace	12
Beet greens, leaves and stems, cooked, drained	1 cup	25	3	Trace	5
Broccoli, cooked, drained:					
Whole stalks, med. size	1 stalk	45	6	1	8
Cut into ½ inch pieces	1 cup	40	5	1	7
Brussels sprouts, 7-8 sprouts per cup, cooked	1 cup	55	7	1	10
Cabbage, common varieties:					
Finely shredded	1 cup	20	1	Trace	5
Cooked	1 cup	30	2	Trace	6
Carrots:					
Raw, whole, 5½ by 1 inch	1 carrot	20	1	Trace	5
Cooked, diced	1 cup	45	1	Trace	10
Cauliflower, cooked, flowerbuds	1 cup	25	3	Trace	5
Celery, raw:					
Stalk, large outer	1 stalk	5	Trace	Trace	2
Pieces, diced	1 cup	15	1	Trace	4
Corn, sweet:					
Cooked, ear 5 by 1¾ inches	1 ear	70	3	1	16
Canned, solids and liquid	1 cup	170	5	2	40
Cucumbers:					
Raw, pared	1 cucumber	30	1	Trace	7

Food	Measure	Food Energy calories*	Protein grams	Fat grams	Carbohydrate grams
Raw, pared, sliced 1/8 inch thick	6 slices	5	Trace	Trace	2
Lettuce, raw	1 head	60	4	Trace	13
Mushrooms, canned, solids and liquid	1 cup	40	5	Trace	6
Onions:					
Mature:					
Raw, 2½ inch diameter	1 onion	40	2	Trace	10
Cooked	1 cup	60	3	Trace	14
Young green, small, without tops	6 onions	20	1	Trace	5
Parsley, raw, chopped	1 tbsp.	Trace	Trace	Trace	Trace
Peas, green, cooked	1 cup	115	9	1	19
Peppers, green, raw	1 pod	15	1	Trace	4
Potatoes, medium (3 per lb., raw):					
Boiled, peeled after boiling	1 potato	105	3	Trace	23
French fried, cooked in deep fat, piece 2 by ½ by ½ inch	10 pieces	155	2	7	20
Mashed, milk added	1 cup	125	4	1	25
Potato chips, medium	10 chips	115	1	8	10
Radishes, raw, small	4 radishes	5	Trace	Trace	1
Sauerkraut, canned, solids and liquid	1 cup	45	2	Trace	9
Spinach, cooked	1 cup	40	5	1	6
Squash, cooked:					
Summer, diced	1 cup	30	2	Trace	7
Winter, baked, mashed	1 cup	130	4	1	32
Sweet potatoes:					

Baked, medium, peeled after baking	1 sweet potato	155	2	1	36
Canned	1 cup	235	4	Trace	54
Tomatoes:					
Raw, wt. 7 oz.	1 tomato	40	2	Trace	9
Canned, solids and liquid	1 cup	50	2	1	10
Tomato catsup	1 tbsp.	15	Trace	Trace	4
Tomato juice	1 cup	45	2	Trace	10

FRUITS AND FRUIT PRODUCTS

Apples, raw (3 per lb.)	1 apple	70	Trace	Trace	18
Apple juice	1 cup	120	Trace	Trace	30
Applesauce, canned, sweetened	1 cup	230	1	Trace	61
Apricots:					
Raw (12 per lb.)	3 apricots	55	1	Trace	14
Canned in heavy syrup	1 cup	220	2	Trace	57
Avocados, whole, raw	1 avocado	370	5	37	13
Bananas, raw, medium size	1 banana	100	1	Trace	26
Blackberries, raw	1 cup	85	2	1	19
Blueberries, raw	1 cup	85	1	1	21
Cantaloupe, raw, medium	½ melon	60	1	Trace	14
Cranberry juice, canned	1 cup	165	Trace	Trace	42
Cranberry sauce, sweetened, canned, strained	1 cup	405	Trace	1	104
Fruit cocktail, canned, in heavy syrup	1 cup	195	1	Trace	50
Grapefruit, raw, medium	½ grapefruit	50	1	Trace	13
Grapefruit juice, canned, unsweetened	1 cup	100	1	Trace	24
Grapes, raw (American type)	1 cup	65	1	1	15
Grapejuice:					

Food	Measure	Food Energy calories*	Protein grams	Fat grams	Carbohydrate grams
Canned or bottled	1 cup	165	1	1	42
Frozen concentrate, sweetened, diluted with 3 parts water, by volume	1 cup	135	1	1	33
Lemon juice, raw	1 cup	60	1	1	20
Lemonade concentrate, diluted with 4-1/3 parts water, by volume	1 cup	110	Trace	Trace	28
Lime juice, fresh or canned, unsweetened	1 cup	65	1	1	22
Oranges, raw, 2½ inch diameter	1 orange	65	1	Trace	16
Orange juice, fresh	1 cup	110	2	2	26
Canned unsweetened or frozen concentrate diluted with 3 parts water, by volume	1 cup	120	2	2	29
Peaches:					
Raw, whole, medium	1 peach	35	1	1	10
Canned, solids and liquid:					
Syrup pack, heavy	1 cup	200	1	1	52
Water pack	1 cup	75	1	1	20
Pears:					
Raw	1 pear	100	1	1	25
Canned, solids and liquid, syrup pack, heavy	1 cup	195	1	1	50
Pineapple:					
Raw, diced	1 cup	75	1	1	19
Canned, heavy syrup pack, solids and liquid:					
Crushed	1 cup	195	1	1	50
Sliced, with juice	1 large slice	90	Trace	Trace	24
Pineapple juice, canned	1 cup	135	1	1	34
Plums, raw	1 plum	25	Trace	Trace	7

Food	Measure				
Prunes, dried, medium	4 prunes	70	1	Trace	18
Prune juice, canned or bottled	1 cup	200	1	Trace	49
Raisins, seedless	1 oz.	80	Trace	Trace	22
Raspberries, red:					
Raw	1 cup	70	1	1	17
Frozen, 10 oz. carton	1 carton	275	2	1	70
Strawberries:					
Raw, capped	1 cup	55	1	1	13
Frozen, 10 oz. carton	1 carton	310	1	1	79
Tangerines, raw, medium	1 tangerine	40	1	Trace	10
Watermelon, raw, wedge, 4 by 8 inches	1 wedge	115	2	1	27

GRAIN PRODUCTS

Food	Measure				
Bagel, 3-inch diameter	1 bagel	165	6	2	28
Barley, pearled, light, uncooked	1 cup	700	16	2	158
Biscuits, baking powder from home recipe, 2-inch diameter	1 biscuit	105	2	5	13
Bran flakes (40% bran)	1 cup	105	4	1	28
Bran flakes with raisins	1 cup	145	4	1	40
Breads:					
Boston brown bread, slice 3 by ¾ inch	1 slice	100	3	1	22
Raisin bread, 18 slices per 1 lb. loaf	1 slice	65	2	1	13
Rye bread, American, light, 18 slices per 1 lb. loaf	1 slice	60	2	Trace	13
White bread, enriched:					
Slice, 18 slices per 1 lb. loaf	1 slice	70	2	1	13
Slice, 22 slices per 1 lb. loaf	1 slice	55	2	1	10
Whole wheat bread, 18 slices per 1 lb. loaf	1 slice	60	3	1	12
Breadcrumbs, dry, grated	1 cup	390	13	5	73
Cakes made from cake mixes:					
Angelfood, 1/12 of 10-inch diameter cake	1 piece	135	3	Trace	32

Food	Measure	Food Energy calories*	Protein grams	Fat grams	Carbohydrate grams
Cupcakes, small, 2½-inch diameter, with chocolate icing	1 cupcake	130	2	5	21
Devil's food, 2-layer, with chocolate icing, 1/16 of 9-inch diameter cake	1 piece	235	3	9	40
Gingerbread, 1/9 of 8-inch square cake	1 piece	175	2	4	32
Cakes made from home recipes:					
Fruitcake, dark, 1/30 of 8-inch loaf	1 slice	55	1	2	9
Pound, slice, ½ inch thick	1 slice	140	2	9	14
Cookies:					
Brownies with nuts, made from home recipe	1 brownie	95	1	6	10
Chocolate chip, commercial	1 cookie	50	1	2	7
Fig bars, commercial	1 cookie	50	1	1	11
Sandwich, chocolate or vanilla, commercial	1 cookie	50	1	2	7
Corn flakes, added nutrients:					
Plain	1 cup	100	2	Trace	21
Sugar-covered	1 cup	155	2	Trace	36
Corn muffins, made with enriched degermed cornmeal and enriched flour; 2½ inch diameter	1 muffin	125	3	4	19
Corn, puffed, presweetened, added nutrients	1 cup	115	1	Trace	27
Crackers:					
Graham, 2½ inch square	4 crackers	110	2	3	21
Saltines	4 crackers	50	1	1	8
Danish pastry, plain round piece, 4½ diameter by 1 inch	1 pastry	175	5	15	30
Doughnuts, cake type	1 doughnut	125	1	6	16
Macaroni, enriched, cooked until tender	1 cup	155	5	1	32
Macaroni (enriched) and cheese, baked	1 cup	430	17	22	40

Muffins, with enriched white flour; 3-inch diameter	1 muffin	120	3	4	17
Noodles (egg noodles), cooked, enriched	1 cup	200	7	2	37
Oatmeal, or rolled oats, cooked	1 cup	130	5	2	23
Pancakes, 4-inch diameter, wheat, plain, or buttermilk	1 cake	60	2	2	9
Pie (piecrust made with unenriched flour); sector, 4-inch, 1/7 of 9-inch diameter pie:					
Apple (2-crust)	1 sector	350	3	15	51
Cherry (2-crust)	1 sector	350	4	15	52
Custard (1-crust)	1 sector	285	8	14	30
Lemon meringue (1-crust)	1 sector	305	4	12	45
Pecan (1-crust)	1 sector	490	6	27	60
Pumpkin (1-crust)	1 sector	275	5	15	32
Pizza (cheese); 1/8 of 14-inch diameter pie	1 sector	185	7	6	27
Popcorn, popped:					
With oil and salt	1 cup	40	1	2	5
Sugar coated	1 cup	135	2	1	30
Pretzels:					
Dutch, twisted	1 pretzel	60	2	1	12
Stick, regular, 3 inch	5 sticks	10	Trace	Trace	2
Rice, white, enriched, cooked	1 cup	225	4	Trace	50
Rice, puffed, added nutrients	1 cup	60	1	Trace	13
Rolls, enriched:					
Cloverleaf or pan, home recipe	1 roll	120	3	3	20
Frankfurter or hamburger	1 roll	120	3	2	21
Rye wafers, whole-grain, 2 by 3½ inches	2 wafers	45	2	Trace	10
Spaghetti, cooked, tender stage, enriched	1 cup	155	5	1	32
Spaghetti with meat balls and tomato sauce, canned	1 cup	260	12	10	28
Waffles, with enriched flour, 7-inch diameter	1 waffle	210	7	7	28
Wheat, puffed, added nutrients	1 cup	55	2	Trace	12
Wheat, shredded, plain	1 biscuit	90	2	1	20
Wheat flakes, added nutrients	1 cup	105	3	Trace	24

Food	Measure	Food Energy calories*	Protein grams	Fat grams	Carbohydrate grams
Wheat flours:					
Whole-wheat, from hard wheats, stirred	1 cup	400	16	2	85
All-purpose or family flour, enriched, sifted	1 cup	420	12	1	88
FATS, OILS					
Butter:					
Regular, 4 sticks per lb.	1 tbsp.	100	Trace	12	Trace
Whipped, 6 sticks or 2 8-oz. containers per lb.	1 tbsp.	65	Trace	8	Trace
Fats, cooking:					
Lard	1 cup	1,850	0	205	0
	1 tbsp.	115	0	13	0
Vegetable fats	1 cup	1,770	0	200	0
	1 tbsp.	110	0	13	0
Margarine, regular, 4 sticks per lb.	1 tbsp.	100	Trace	12	Trace
Oils, salad or cooking (corn, cottonseed, olive, peanut, safflower, soybean)	1 cup	1,945	0	220	0
	1 tbsp.	125	0	14	0
Salad dressings:					
Blue cheese	1 tbsp.	75	1	8	1
Commercial, mayonnaise type	1 tbsp.	65	Trace	6	2
French	1 tbsp.	65	Trace	6	3
Mayonnaise	1 tbsp.	100	Trace	11	Trace
Thousand island	1 tbsp.	80	Trace	8	3

SUGARS, SWEETS

Candy:					
Caramels, plain or chocolate	1 oz.	115	1	3	22
Chocolate, milk, plain	1 oz.	145	2	9	16
Fudge, plain	1 oz.	115	1	4	21
Hard	1 oz.	110	0	Trace	28
Chocolate-flavored syrup or topping:					
Thin type	1 fl. oz.	90	1	1	24
Fudge type	1 fl. oz.	125	2	5	20
Chocolate-flavored beverage powder, without nonfat dry milk (approx. 4 heaping tsp. per oz.)	1 oz.	100	1	1	25
Honey, strained or extracted	1 tbsp.	65	Trace	0	17
Jams and preserves	1 tbsp.	55	Trace	Trace	14
Jellies	1 tbsp.	50	Trace	Trace	13
Molasses, cane:					
Light (first extraction)	1 tbsp.	50	Trace	Trace	13
Blackstrap (third extraction)	1 tbsp.	45	Trace	Trace	11
Syrup, table blends, chiefly corn, light and dark	1 tbsp.	60	0	0	15
Sugar, white, granulated	1 tbsp.	40	0	0	11

MISCELLANEOUS ITEMS

Beverages, alcoholic:					
Beer	12 fl. oz.	150	1	0	14
Gin, rum, vodka, whiskey:					
86-proof	1½ fl. oz. (jigger)	105	Trace	Trace	Trace
100-proof	1½ fl. oz. (jigger)	125	Trace	Trace	Trace

Food	Measure	Food Energy calories*	Protein grams	Fat grams	Carbohydrate grams
Wines:					
Dessert	3½ fl. oz. glass	140	Trace	0	8
Table	3½ fl. oz. glass	85	Trace	0	4
Beverages, carbonated, sweetened, nonalcoholic::					
Carbonated water	12 fl. oz.	115	0	0	29
Cola type	12 fl. oz.	145	0	0	37
Fruit-flavored sodas and Tom Collins mixes	12 fl. oz.	170	0	0	45
Root beer	12 fl. oz.	150	0	0	39
Bouillon cubes, ½ inch	1 cube	5	1	Trace	Trace
Chocolate, bitter or baking	1 oz.	145	3	15	8
Gelatin, plain, dry powder in envelope	1 envelope	25	6	Trace	0
Gelatin dessert, prepared with water	1 cup	140	4	0	34
Olives, pickled:					
Green	4 medium	15	Trace	2	Trace
Ripe: Mission	3 small	15	Trace	2	Trace
Pickles, cucumber:					
Dill, medium, whole	1 pickle	10	1	Trace	1
Sweet, gherkin, small, whole	1 pickle	20	Trace	Trace	6
Relish, finely chopped, sweet	1 tbsp.	20	Trace	Trace	5
Pudding, home recipe with starch base:					
Chocolate	1 cup	385	8	12	67
Vanilla (blanc mange)	1 cup	285	9	10	41

Sherbet	1 cup	260	2	2	59
Soups, canned, condensed, ready-to-serve:					
Prepared with an equal volume of milk:					
Cream of chicken	1 cup	180	7	10	15
Cream of mushroom	1 cup	215	7	14	16
Tomato	1 cup	175	7	7	23
Prepared with an equal volume of water:					
Beef broth, bouillon, consomme	1 cup	30	5	0	3
Beef noodle	1 cup	70	4	3	7
Cream of chicken	1 cup	95	3	6	8
Cream of mushroom	1 cup	135	2	10	10
Minestrone	1 cup	105	5	3	14
Split pea	1 cup	145	9	3	21
Tomato	1 cup	90	2	3	16
Vegetable beef	1 cup	80	5	2	10
Tapioca desserts:					
Apple	1 cup	295	1	Trace	74
Cream pudding	1 cup	220	8	8	28
Tartar sauce	1 tbsp.	75	Trace	8	1
Vinegar	1 tbsp.	Trace	Trace	0	1
White sauce, medium	1 cup	405	10	31	22

*The Calorie used in human metabolism is the heat needed to raise the temperature of one kilogram (2.2 pounds) of water from 15 degrees to 16 degrees Centigrade.

Adapted from U. S. Department of Agriculture, Agricultural Research Service, *Nutritive value of foods.* (Home and Garden Bulletin No. 72) Washington, D.C.: U. S. Government Printing Office, 1970.

APPENDIX F

MEAN ENERGY EXPENDITURE OF VARIOUS ACTIVITIES

The values are expressed in calories/minute of gross body expenditure.

	Body weight, pounds	Calories*/ minute
1. Personal necessities		
Sitting, eating	143	1.5
Sleeping	150	1.2
Washing and dressing	150	2.6
2. Locomotion		
Cycling, 5.5 mph	156	4.5
Cycling, 9.4 mph	156	7.0
Cycling, 13.1 mph	156	11.1
Driving a car	141	2.8
Walking, 2 mph	160	3.2
Walking, 3 mph	160	4.4
Walking, 4 mph	160	5.8
Walking downstairs	161	7.1
Walking upstairs	161	18.6
3. Sedentary occupations		
Classwork, lecture	150	1.7
Sitting, reading	161	1.3
Standing, light activity	161	2.6
Typing, 40 words/min., mechanical typewriter	121	1.7
Typing, 40 words/min., electric typewriter	121	1.5
4. Domestic work		
Bed making	121	3.5
Dusting	121	2.5
Ironing	121	1.7
Preparing a meal	121	2.5
Scrubbing floors	121	4.0
Shopping with heavy load	121	4.0
Window cleaning	121	3.5
5. Light industry		
Assembly work in car factory	121	2.3
Carpentry	150	3.8
Farming chores	150	3.8
Farming, haying, plowing with horse	150	6.7
House painting	150	3.5
Metal working	150	3.5
Mixing cement	150	4.7
Stone, masonry	150	6.3
Truck and automobile repair	150	4.2

6. Heavy work

Dragging logs	143	12.1
Drilling coal or rock	143	6.1
Felling trees	143	8.6
Gardening, digging	139	8.6
Pick and shovel work	143	8.6

7. Recreation

Canoeing, 2.5 mph	150	3.0
Canoeing, 4 mph	150	7.0
Cross country running	143	10.6
Dancing, waltz	167	5.2
Dancing, rumba	152	5.7
Golfing	139	5.0
Gymnastics exercises:		
Balancing exercises	150	2.5
Trunk bending	150	3.5
Mountain climbing	150	10.0
Playing baseball (except pitcher)	150	4.7
Playing basketball	161	8.6
Playing football (American)	161	10.2
Playing pingpong	161	4.9
Playing tennis	154	7.1
Playing squash	147	10.2
Playing volleyball	150	3.5
Skiing, level hard snow, moderate speed	125	10.8
Skiing, up hill hard snow, maximum speed	150	18.6
Sprinting	150	23.3
Snowshoeing 2.27 mph	150	6.2

*The calorie used in human metabolism is the heat needed to raise the temperature of one kilogram (2.2 pounds) of water from 15 degrees to 16 degrees Centigrade.

Adapted from the following:
J. V. G. A. Durnin and R. Passmore, *Energy, work and leisure.* London: Heinemann Educational Books Ltd., 1967. Pp. 49, 57, 72, 76.

R. Passmore and J. V. G. A. Durnin, Human energy expenditure, *Physiological Reviews*, 1955, *35*, 811-813.

C. F. Consolazio, R. E. Johnson, and L. J. Pecora, *Physiological measurements of metabolic functions in man.* New York. McGraw-Hill, 1963. Pp. 330-332.

DAILY EATING, EXERCISE, AND WEIGHT GRAPH

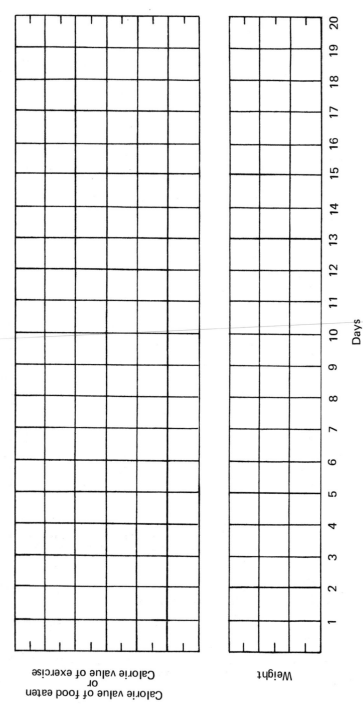

Calorie value of food eaten
or
Calorie value of exercise

Weight

Days

1 2 3 4 5 6 7 8 9 10 11 12 13 14 15 16 17 18 19 20

DAILY EATING, EXERCISE, AND WEIGHT GRAPH

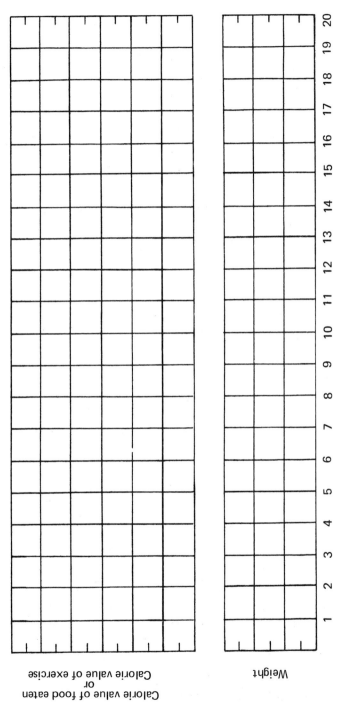

Calorie value of food eaten
or
Calorie value of exercise

Weight

Days

DAILY EATING, EXERCISE, AND WEIGHT GRAPH

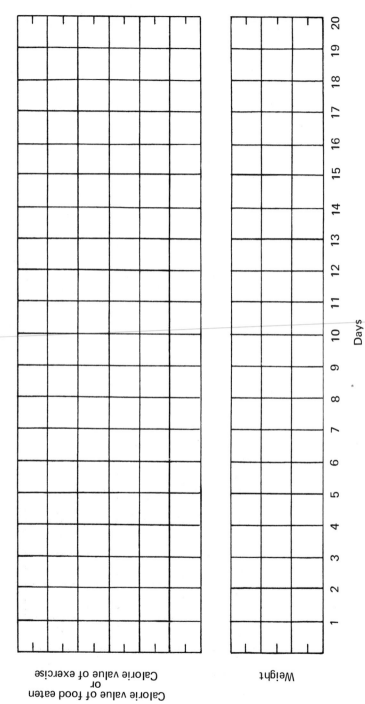

Calorie value of food eaten
or
Calorie value of exercise

Weight

Days

1　2　3　4　5　6　7　8　9　10　11　12　13　14　15　16　17　18　19　20

240

DAILY EATING, EXERCISE, AND WEIGHT GRAPH

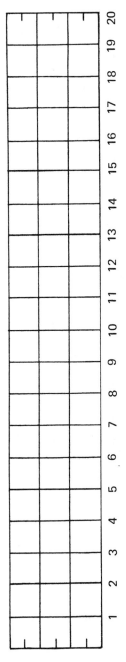

Calorie value of food eaten
or
Calorie value of exercise

Weight

Days

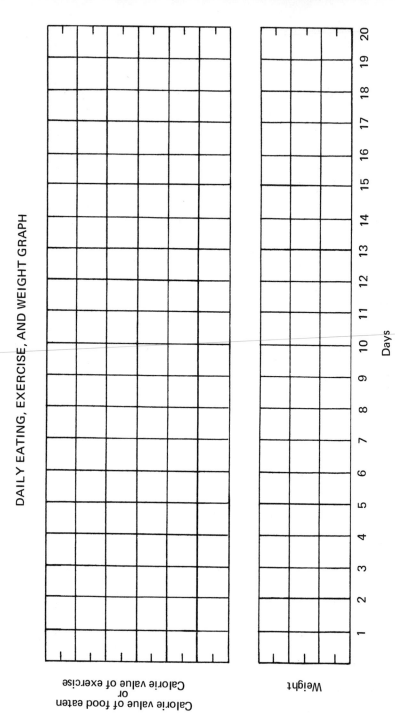

DAILY EATING, EXERCISE, AND WEIGHT GRAPH

Calorie value of food eaten
or
Calorie value of exercise

Weight

Days

1 2 3 4 5 6 7 8 9 10 11 12 13 14 15 16 17 18 19 20

DAILY EATING, EXERCISE, AND WEIGHT GRAPH

Calorie value of food eaten
or
Calorie value of exercise

Weight

Days

1 2 3 4 5 6 7 8 9 10 11 12 13 14 15 16 17 18 19 20

243

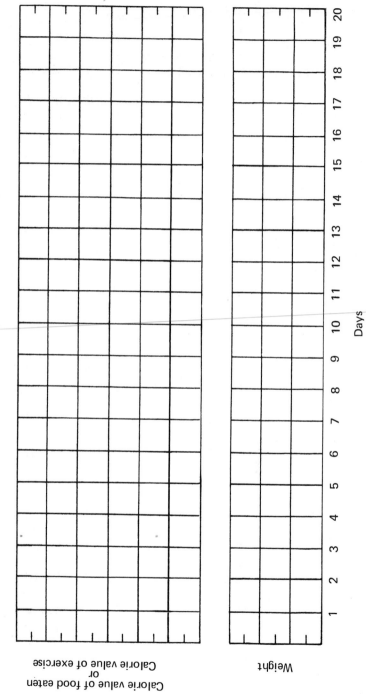

DAILY EATING, EXERCISE, AND WEIGHT GRAPH

Calorie value of food eaten
or
Calorie value of exercise

Weight

Days

1 2 3 4 5 6 7 8 9 10 11 12 13 14 15 16 17 18 19 20

DAILY EATING, EXERCISE, AND WEIGHT GRAPH

Calorie value of food eaten
or
Calorie value of exercise

Weight

Days

1 2 3 4 5 6 7 8 9 10 11 12 13 14 15 16 17 18 19 20

245